Praise for *PCOS SOS Fertility Fast Track*

"Dr. Gersh brings much-needed clarity, sanity, and optimism to the world of PCOS infertility. Her practical 12-week program optimizes the health of mothers-to-be so they have their best chances of getting pregnant and having the babies they so badly yearn for. If you are a woman with PCOS who wants to have a baby, you need to read Dr. Gersh's incredible book!"

~ JJ Virgin,
New York Times bestselling author of *The Virgin Diet*

"In her latest groundbreaking book, PCOS SOS Fertility Fast Track, Dr. Gersh provides a powerful, all-natural treatment plan for the infertility suffered by so many PCOS women. With her characteristic warmth, clarity, and practicality, Dr. Gersh makes both healthy living and the science behind it accessible and easy to understand. Fertility and reproduction are transformative experiences that are frequently denied to women with PCOS. Dr. Gersh shows women how, in 12 weeks, they can reclaim their health and fertility so they have the best chance to get pregnant and give birth to the children they yearn for. If you are a woman with PCOS and you want to have a baby, read this book!"

~ Naomi Whittel,
New York Times bestselling author of *Glow 15*

"There is no better doctor and teacher than Felice Gersh, M.D. when it comes to women's health, hormone issues, and polycystic ovary syndrome. There are very few people we meet throughout life who truly change lives. Dr. Gersh is one of those people. Every woman should read this book."

~Nathan S. Bryan, Ph.D.,
Baylor College of Medicine

"Dr. Gersh's new fertility book will undoubtedly result in many new babies coming into the world!"

~Lara Briden, N.D.,
bestselling author of the *Period Repair Manual*

"Dr Gersh lays out a simple but comprehensive explanation of PCOS and gives women a blueprint for how to take control of their health and fertility. Her three-month preconception plan is a highly worthwhile investment for any couple that wants a low-risk pregnancy and a healthy baby."

~**Dr. Jim Parker, OB/GYN**
and Endoscopic Surgeon, Nutritional and
Environmental Medicine Health Researcher

"As a gynecologist who treats thousands of women with PCOS, Dr. Felice Gersh is certainly the absolute authority on the subject. She brings clarity and concise direction to such a confusing and overwhelming issue that many women are diagnosed with. I highly recommend her book and it is something that I want every PCOS patient to read."

~**Dr. Anna Cabeca, D.O., FACOG, ABAARM, ABoIM**
and bestselling author of *The Hormone Fix*

"PCOS SOS *Fertility Fast Track* is a must-read for every woman with PCOS who dreams of holding her healthy baby, following a complication free pregnancy. This 12-week program offers a clear path to optimized fertility.

~**Robyn Openshaw, MSW,**
founder of GreenSmoothieGirl.com and bestselling author of *Vibe*

"PCOS is not a fertility death sentence. It is simply an endocrine difference. In her book PCOS SOS *Fertility Fast Track*, Dr. Gersh exquisitely outlines a clear roadmap to optimal health, which increases every PCOS woman's odds of getting pregnant, staying pregnant, and experiencing the incredible joys of motherhood. While a typical PCOS diagnosis is ladened with doom and gloom, Dr. Gersh takes a different approach. Because she has a clear understanding of this endocrine difference, her treatment recommendations burst with hope. In our opinion, every person who has been diagnosed with or thinks they may have PCOS needs this book."

~**Dr. Mark Sherwood, N.D. & Dr. Michele Neil-Sherwood, D.O.,**
bestselling authors of *Quest for Wellness, Fork Your Diet,*
and Surviving the *Garden of Eatin'*; executive producers of
the Amazon hit healthumentary movie, *Fork Your Diet*

"PCOS SOS *Fertility Fast Track* is a fresh take on how to manage PCOS. I believe that Dr. Gersh is probably the only doctor in the United States who has 40 plus years of clinical experience as a gynaecologist treating women with PCOS combined with a board-certification in Integrative Medicine. This unique synergy allows Dr. Gersh to offer innovative advice on a huge array of non-traditional therapies for managing the various clinical concerns of PCOS, particularly infertility and pregnancy complications. As such, her book offers new hope to women with PCOS who want to become mothers. I am proud to call Dr. Gersh a friend and consider her an inspiration for advancing medical care in women's health."

~Kelton Tremellen, M.D., PhD,
Professor of Reproductive Medicine, Adelaide, South Australia

PCOS SOS
Fertility
Fast Track

The 12 Week Plan To
Optimize Your Chances Of

A Successful Pregnancy

And A Healthy Baby

Felice Gersh, M.D.
with Alexis Perella

Health Disclaimer

This book contains advice and information relating to health care. It should be used to supplement rather than replace the advice of your doctor or another trained health professional. If you know or suspect you have a health problem, it is recommended that you seek your physician's advice before embarking on any medical program or treatment. All efforts have been made to assure the accuracy of the information contained in this book as of the date of publication. The publisher and the author disclaim liability for any medical outcome that may occur as a result of applying the methods suggested in this book.

Printed in the United States
First printing, 2019

ISBN (paperback) 978-1-950634-02-6
ISBN (eBook) 978-1-950634-03-3

Integrative Medical Press
4968 Booth Circle, Suite 101
Irvine, CA 92604
United States of America

Dedication

*D*r. Walter Crinnion was my brilliant and caring teacher, influential colleague, and close friend.

Always decades ahead of the pack, Dr. Crinnion was one of the pioneers of environmental medicine and his was one of the first voices to warn against the dangers of the ubiquitous industrial chemicals that we are all exposed to daily. I was incredibly lucky to learn environmental medicine from him. Without a doubt, his passion and dedication to understanding how small exposures to environmental chemicals could have profound impacts on the human body shaped me into the doctor I am today. Walter demonstrated that plastics and plasticizers, flame retardants, water repellents, heavy metals, pesticides, and herbicides damage the human immune system, lead to chronic inflammation and sometimes chronic infections, dysregulate metabolic health, and ultimately reduce female fertility. Always a pragmatic optimist, Walter guided me to seek solutions for my patients impacted by environmental toxins and advised me as I developed strategies to help all of my patients reduce their exposures.

Dr. Crinnion started out as my teacher, but after I graduated from his classes, we became colleagues. I was honored to lecture and teach alongside him, especially at the fantastic annual Environmental Healthcare Symposium that he put on with Dr. Lyn Patrick.

While working together, Walter and I quickly became friends. We saw eye to eye on so many topics. We began planning to one day write a book together about the effects of environmental pollution on women's health.

Tragically, Dr. Crinnion recently passed away, far too young and much too early.

Dear friend, I miss your humor, amazing kindness, and astute wisdom.

To you, Walter, I dedicate my book, for without the time we shared, I doubt this book would have come to be written.

With deepest gratitude,
Felice

Contents

Foreword by Sara Gottfried, M.D.

*I*f you've been struggling with polycystic ovary syndrome (PCOS) and fertility, this book may be exactly what you need. When given a PCOS diagnosis, many women feel like they cannot trust their body anymore, but that's simply not true. As Felice Gersh, M.D. shows directly and cogently, PCOS is a normal human variation. It's been around for generations and didn't always result in medical extremes, such as infertility. PCOS is a condition that gets exaggerated by lifestyle and environmental influences, and this is what leads to health and fertility problems.

I've been in that place of uncertainty, unsure whether I could trust my own body, and maybe you have, too. I have battled insulin resistance, and while many members of my family have been diagnosed with PCOS, I do not personally carry the diagnosis, although I suspect I am a borderline case. I have prediabetes, acne, and hirsutism. More troubling, I have had persistent weight gain coupled with weight loss resistance, particularly after the birth of my daughters. The only solutions offered by my mainstream doctor were to exercise more, eat less, and take a birth control pill. Those options left me cold, because they didn't address the root cause of my symptoms, nor did they honor the wisdom of my female body.

I applied my medical knowledge to myself and found a way to reset my hormones with the way I eat, think, move, and supplement—and wrote a few bestselling books about it. I became a believer in the power of lifestyle redesign as the best medicine. At first, my beliefs set me apart from other physicians who clung to their pharmaceuticals as the only option. It was lonely. Over time, I looked for similar-minded physicians and other clinicians and built bridges with them. But nothing prepared me for the connection I felt with Dr. Gersh.

Dr. Gersh and I had been connected for years through a Bay Area Functional Medicine group. This year, we were asked to co-teach a course on women's health at a national conference in Florida. As I sat in the audience and witnessed Dr. Gersh, a fellow board-certified obstetrician/gynecologist, talk about the breadth and depth of the health issues women face, something inside of me clicked. Over decades of busy medical practice, hundreds of miles apart, we had arrived at so many of the same conclusions, foundational approaches, and beliefs about being in tune with our bodies and aligned with nature. Estrogen is the master regulator of the female body. Insulin and testosterone get out of whack with common lifestyle choices. We even agree on the best food-first approaches to solve these problems, although nutrition can be as controversial as politics.

Bringing a new life into this world may be the greatest joy you'll know. While it may or may not be something you choose or experience, what I most hope for you is that you have the option—that you have access to well-proven strategies that can help you get pregnant, experience a healthy gestation and delivery, and heal and reconstitute postpartum. Few conventional obstetrician/gynecologists know about the basic nutritional and lifestyle interventions that are proven to reverse PCOS, infertility, gestational diabetes, and even preterm labor.

Typically when women go to the doctor's office with fertility problems, the wisdom of their bodies get neglected. They are pushed into risky and invasive procedures, all with the goal of getting a positive pregnancy test—not a healthy baby or mom. This approach ignores the conditions that contributed to problems with fertility, and it overlooks the health of the mom-to-be and what those problematic conditions might mean to her developing baby. This is like cutting the wire to your "check engine" light instead of finding and fixing the real problem with your car—sounds kind of short-sighted, doesn't it?

Yes, we can trick your body into ovulating; we can fertilize several eggs and implant them in your uterus. One (or more) may develop to full-term, and you'll have a baby (or several), but at what cost? No, I'm not just talking about the tens of thousands of dollars you'll pay out-of-pocket for fertility treatments. What will be the health cost to you and your baby? In this book, Dr. Gersh tells you exactly why these risky and invasive procedures should be sought only as a last resort, after you've taken care of your own health and managed your PCOS, not before.

In regards to PCOS, pregnancy, and birth, Dr. Gersh is an expert in the field. She has over 40 years in practice. She's seen it all, and even to an experienced gynecologist like myself, she's the kind of woman you turn to for guidance. She graduated from Princeton University before earning her medical degree from the University of Southern California (USC). She went on to teach surgery to new doctors at USC. She has seen not only where modern medicine has advanced, but also where it's failed her patients. Because of these limitations, she sought answers for patients who were struggling to get pregnant or experienced problems during their pregnancies. After decades in practice, Dr. Gersh knew there was more than the conventional medical model was teaching her. Instead of resting on her laurels, she completed a fellowship in Integrative Medicine at the University of Arizona's prestigious Andrew Weil Center, making her one of the extremely rare doctors who is double board-certified in Obstetrics/Gynecology and Integrative Medicine. When it comes to understanding PCOS and how to get women pregnant with personalized lifestyle medicine, Dr. Gersh is the fertility goddess!

PCOS has far-ranging consequences on your health beyond just getting pregnant, although we know that's why you picked up this book. Dr. Gersh's PCOS SOS Fertility Fast Track protocol will help you to understand that PCOS is a condition that affects your whole body, not just your ovaries. The term PCOS is confusing for patients and doctors alike; the syndrome can't just be boiled down to small cysts in the ovaries. Dr. Gersh will help you to understand what it means to have PCOS, how it's a normal variation that affects your blood sugar and hormones, and why, when your lifestyle steps on the gas pedal of these variations, it causes (often reversible) infertility. She will teach you the value of food, lifestyle, and targeted natural supplements as medicine. She will help you change your lifestyle and health in 12 weeks.

This book will guide you, step-by-step, to getting your body ready for a healthy pregnancy. In my own OB/GYN practice I've used the techniques Dr. Gersh describes in this book and have been astonished by how many beautiful, naturally pregnant women come into my exam rooms, beaming with happiness—usually after being told by other doctors their only choice for getting pregnant was in vitro fertilization (IVF). These pregnancies didn't "just happen" because our patients were lucky. As their doctors, we looked deep into the science of why they weren't getting pregnant, and these patients put forth solid efforts to get themselves healthy enough to get pregnant. And you know what else? These women consistently tell us that the process of going through the PCOS SOS Fertility Fast Track helped prepare them for being a parent. Let Dr. Gersh help show you a better way to getting pregnant with PCOS.

The transcendent feeling of supporting a new mother as she delivers a beautiful new baby drove Dr. Gersh and me to become obstetrician/ gynecologists and, ultimately, mothers. We want you to have a healthy pregnancy and baby—and to progress through these major lifecycle transitions with great dignity, autonomy, and education. We want you and your baby to go home without visiting the hospital's operating room or neonatal intensive care units (NICU). Dr. Gersh and I have helped tens of thousands of women welcome their new babies into the world. These are the peak experiences in our work: Witnessing a new mom embracing her newborn in the first moments of life puts everything else in perspective.

Dr. Gersh is a seasoned expert in our shared field of women's health. You probably cannot find a better guide on this highly personal, physically and emotionally demanding journey.

Sara Gottfried, M.D.
Berkeley, California

Foreword by Lyn Patrick, N.D.

*F*elice, every time we meet, I am struck by how much you remind me of one of my all-time heroes of environmental health, Dr. Theo Colborn. She was an outspoken adversary of industrial polluters, especially the oil and gas industry. She helped coin the term "endocrine disruptors," she testified to the U.S. government about the need for natural gas companies to disclose the chemicals used in production, and she spent countless hours educating the public about topics such as water contamination caused by fracking and linking it to cancer clusters.

You and Theo both have the same fearless energy and commitment to discovering and sharing truth, even when it's not popular, even when you risk making enemies of powerful corporations. Where she challenged industrial polluters, you challenge pharmaceutical companies. You have both advocated your causes to the U.S. government. You both have given innumerable hours of your time to educating people around the world.

Additionally, you both have the same brilliance. You are able to look at research and see the deepest implications. At the same time, you can recognize what is missing and what remains to be done.

I will always remember Dr. Theo Colborn for the way she changed the discussion around environmental exposures and endocrine disruptors.

Felice, you are in the prime of producing your most significant work so I wouldn't want to bestow your legacy too soon. But I suspect it will have something to do with the effects of lifestyle and environmental exposures on female reproduction. Or perhaps it will revolve more generally around endocrine disruptors and female hormones. Or, perhaps in the coming years, you will participate in more groundbreaking discoveries that we have yet to foresee.

Already, I have learned so much from you about using natural therapies such as sleep hygiene, nutrition, intermittent fasting, estrogen optimization, support for the gut microbiome, and exercise to treat PCOS, infertility, and many other conditions that women are challenged with today.

I feel privileged to be your friend and to have a front row seat to the incredible work that you are doing. It is my hope that everyone will take advantage of the wisdom in this revolutionary book. Whatever your ultimate legacy ends up being, as with Dr. Theo Colborn, I know many lives will be influenced for the better.

Lyn Patrick, N.D.
Southwestern Colorado

Preface

*O*ver the course of my career, I have spent innumerable hours learning about PCOS and the unique physical and emotional challenges that PCOS women face. Throughout the last decade, I have read every study on PCOS and PCOS-related conditions that has been released. Because PCOS research is grossly underfunded, I have traveled to Washington, D.C. several times to speak with members of the United States Congress, advocating for more resources for PCOS awareness and science. I have been privileged to work with leading scientists to help develop groundbreaking PCOS studies.

With this knowledge and experience, I have formulated cutting edge treatment programs for my own patients with PCOS. Every day, I am privileged to show women how to harness their bodies' capacity for health and healing through lifestyle, supplements, circadian rhythm, and diet, relying on evidence-based natural therapies as first-line treatments and only using pharmaceuticals and more invasive procedures to heal whatever lingering symptoms remain.

The absolute most rewarding part of my medical practice is when I can help a woman with PCOS who was struggling with infertility get pregnant and give birth to a healthy baby.

This is more than an interest or even a passion. It is an undeniable calling and responsibility.

My journey as a PCOS doctor began with my own PCOS story.

When I was six, I got a Tiny Tears baby doll. She could "cry real tears" when she wanted you to hold and feed her! I had a baby stroller, receiving blankets, and all the accoutrements a little girl needed to care for her baby doll. I took that doll everywhere.

I loved her with all of my six-year-old heart and I knew that someday, I wanted to be a real mom with a real baby.

I grew up, as all six-year-olds do. I got married and I went to medical school. And I began to think about having my first baby.

I'd had irregular periods and severe acne since high school, and I'd been on and off birth control pills since early college. I hated those pills with a vengeance because they made me nauseous, but they were the only thing that helped. I'd take the pills for a couple of months, and when I couldn't stand it anymore, I'd quit. And several months later, I'd start all over again.

In those days, Polycystic Ovary Syndrome (PCOS) was called Stein-Leventhal Syndrome, and to get a diagnosis, in addition to having irregular periods, you had to be really obese and practically have a beard. I was relatively small and only had a few easy-to-pluck hairs on my chin. So, I never got a diagnosis beyond "acne and irregular periods."

My husband, Bob, and I decided that we'd try to start our family as soon as I graduated from medical school. I didn't share our plans with anyone, even my mom, because everyone said, "Wait until after residency." But I knew I had fertility problems, and Bob and I wanted several children. I was too scared to wait.

If all worked out as planned, I would be pregnant during my first year of residency in OB-GYN. I have always loved clichés, so I lived by the mantra, "Where there's a will, there's a way!"

But not everyone shared this rosy view.

When I applied for my OB-GYN residency, I was an early female pioneer venturing into what was then a male-dominated career. During my interviews, the one question every program asked, which would be totally illegal now, was "When are you going to have kids?"

I marveled that, although I was applying to care for women's reproductive health, my own female reproductive potential was universally viewed as a negative. So, I did the only thing I could. I lied.

I said, "Someday I'd like to have kids, but I have no current plans."

While I don't generally advocate lying, in this case, it worked out. I was excited to land my number one choice—Kaiser Hospital in Los Angeles.

I spent the first year of my residency delivering the babies of other women. I felt their happiness and celebrated their growing families. When a woman had a pregnancy loss, I gently guided her through the process and shared in her mourning. I loved caring for pregnant women. I loved supporting and shepherding them through this miraculous journey.

But I did not get pregnant that year.

Sometimes, on the weekends, I'd go to the local mall with my husband, and all I could see were babies and toddlers everywhere! I imagined walking up and down the brightly lit walkways with a tiny hand in mine, little feet slapping the tiles. I passed by Bergstrom's baby store and felt the emptiness of my arms.

By the end of that year, I knew it would take more than hope and longing to get pregnant. It had been six months since my last period.

There were only two women attending faculty OB-GYNs at Kaiser. Because I was trying to keep my pregnancy plans a secret, they were the only ones I would see. At the time, it meant so much to me that they helped me without judgment.

I began taking Clomid to induce ovulation. I started at the normal recommended dose, but it didn't work. Nothing happened. So my doctors increased my dosage. Nothing!

I panicked. At this time, there weren't a lot of other options. I could feel my six-year-old self's dreams of a baby slipping away.

My doctors kept me calm. They told me that some women were Clomid-resistant, but sometimes, with a higher dose, they could overcome that resistance. So we tried again and again.

On the sixth try, taking twice the starting dose of Clomid, I got my miracle positive pregnancy test. My husband and I sobbed with joy in each other's arms.

At Kaiser, I refused to let anyone treat me differently. Because I didn't want to miss out on learning and training opportunities, no matter how big and uncomfortable I got, I never complained or missed work. I felt like I had to prove to all the men I worked with that a woman could have babies and continue to practice medicine. I'd never seen another woman do this, so I just did it. I was incredibly lucky that my pregnancy was uncomplicated.

My belly grew at an impossible rate. I got so enormous I could barely wrap my arms around my own stomach. I kept asking my doctors, "Should I be this big? Is this baby huge?" It seemed obvious to me that I was growing a super-sized baby, but no one else seemed worried.

I worked up until the day I delivered. When I went into labor, I pushed and pushed. And when my baby girl finally emerged, she was a shocking nine pounds!

My tiny five foot and an inch body was not made to birth a nine pound baby. I had a fourth degree tear—a rip from vagina to rectum. I am forever indebted to my excellent obstetrician who repaired the wound perfectly.

Baby Alexis was too large to fit into the newborn outfit I'd purchased for the journey home from the hospital. None of the snaps would close!

So we brought her home in a tight tee-shirt, a diaper, and a receiving blanket!

I had always believed that health wasn't a pill. Clomid was hard on me, physically and emotionally. So, after my first baby, I dedicated myself to wellness.

I didn't really know how to eat healthy, but I figured that vegetables were probably important. Never a great cook, I served some kind of steamed veggie with every dinner. And I tried to stay physically active over the following years. I even coached my daughter's pee-wee soccer team and ran up and down the field during practices and games, despite never having played a day of soccer in my life!

I wasn't perfect, but I could tell that I was healthier. For the first time since high school, I had clear, beautiful skin and my periods became regular. Without any additional fertility treatments, I had three more babies.

But I didn't cure my PCOS. In fact, I know now that PCOS is not a disease that can be cured. Rather, I learned to manage it.

It was hard and imperfect. I always joked that I could gain weight just by looking at a donut. And even though I could get pregnant easily after my first, I knew I was still insulin resistant because my babies always came out huge. My middle daughter was the largest, weighing in at a hefty nine pounds, six ounces.

My personal success in controlling PCOS with diet and lifestyle inspired me to look beyond pharmaceuticals to help my many patients with PCOS. What began as my own private story became the focus of my medical career.

When I retired from obstetrics, I went back to school and received my board certification in Integrative Medicine. I learned how diseases and symptoms throughout the body intersect, and I began to research PCOS from a wide range of disciplines. I read about hormones, metabolism, and inflammation. I learned about the importance of estrogen and about

PCOS's tie to insulin resistance. I delved into the gut microbiome. I read article after article on the importance of circadian rhythm and the impact of endocrine disrupting chemicals.

I put all of these pieces together and created my first program to help my PCOS patients get healthy and pregnant. And they did!

Some of my patients had been trying for years. Many of them had been through rounds of failed IVF. After following my protocol, most of my patients got pregnant naturally. Some of them still needed fertility treatments, but suddenly these fertility treatments worked.

Helping women with PCOS get pregnant has become one of the greatest joys of my career. It's something I could have never imagined back when I was desperately, secretly doing round after round of Clomid.

I wrote this book with my eldest daughter, Alexis, who is now a grown woman with children of her own. My goal is to give as many PCOS women as possible their best chance to get pregnant and give birth to healthy babies the way I did and the way my daughter did.

This PCOS SOS Fertility Fast Track program offers more than hope. It is a real and tested path to improve your chances of having the healthy baby you long for.

Female fertility is a sign of female health. Consequently, this program improves fertility by improving all aspects of your health. It is a fast-paced, rigorous program because I'm assuming that if you are here reading this book, then you want to heal your PCOS and your fertility as quickly as possible.

I created this 12-week program for you, to give you a path out of PCOS and into true health and fertility.

I wish you wellness, success, and joy in life, with a hefty sprinkling of baby dust. May the tiny feet that patter through your dreams find a home in your womb, and may you someday hold your dream baby in your arms.

Introduction

*I*f you have PCOS and you want to have a baby, you are in the right place.

Pregnancy is Mother Nature's ultimate stress test for the female body. When you are healthy, you will find it easier to get pregnant. And equally important, when you are healthy, you are more likely to have a healthy pregnancy and give birth to a healthy baby.

That's what this book is about: healthy women and healthy babies.

Consequently, the goal of this book is not to get you pregnant today. The goal is to get you ready for pregnancy so that you have the best chance to conceive naturally and have a safe pregnancy that leads to the full-term birth of a beautiful baby.

As a doctor, I have this goal for every one of my PCOS patients who wants to get pregnant.

Now, I totally understand that if you are reading this book, you probably want to get pregnant *now*. I've been there. I have PCOS, too, and it took me many rounds of fertility treatments to get pregnant with my first baby. Each of those empty attempts was excruciating. Every day, I wanted to be pregnant *now*.

But the truth is, if you have PCOS, the pregnancy odds are stacked against you.

As many as 80% of women with PCOS experience some degree of infertility. And once we get pregnant, we have higher rates of miscarriage and pregnancy complications. Our babies are more likely to spend time in the neonatal intensive care unit (NICU). And if our baby is a girl, she is more likely to develop PCOS when she grows up.[1,2,3]

These are the risks that come with PCOS. But these risks are not insurmountable; they are certainly not destiny. Through smart choices and behaviors, you can dramatically lower these risks and increase your odds of having a safe, successful pregnancy that culminates in the uncomplicated birth of a healthy baby.

A "get-ready-for-pregnancy" book

Typically, when a woman struggles to conceive, the medical community jumps into action, trying to get her pregnant as quickly as possible. She's prescribed fertility drugs, such as Clomid, to trick her body into ovulating. If she is overweight, she's offered an extremely restrictive diet to help her lose weight as rapidly and dramatically as possible. If these efforts don't result in conception, she will embark on a path of increasingly invasive and expensive procedures—additional fertility drugs, surgical interventions such as ovarian drilling, intrauterine insemination, in-vitro fertilization—all aimed at getting to that positive pregnancy test.

And what then? She is transferred to more medical specialists to monitor her now high-risk pregnancy in the hopes that she avoids complications and stays pregnant long enough for her baby to be safely delivered.

Yes, there is a place for all of these treatments. But often, doctors turn to these treatments as first-line therapies when they should really be last resorts.

Pregnancies achieved through any form of Assisted Reproductive Technology (ART) are not as safe for mother and baby as naturally occurring pregnancies. The risks differ depending on the specific fertility treatment, but across the board, all ART pregnancies have higher rates of miscarriage, preeclampsia, gestational diabetes, placenta previa, placental abruption, cesarean section, preterm delivery, and stillbirth.[4]

Part of the problem is that a significant percentage of ART pregnancies are multiples (twins, occasionally triplets, and sometimes even more) and these are always riskier than singleton pregnancies. But that's not the only factor. When we compare natural singleton pregnancies and IVF singleton pregnancies, IVF pregnancies are associated with more pregnancy complications and poorer outcomes, including higher rates of maternal and fetal death.[5,6]

Not only are ART pregnancies riskier, ART is expensive. And often, the treatments are not covered by insurance.

Of course, I'm not saying that we should never use these treatments, but they shouldn't be the default. Not when most women can greatly enhance their fertility naturally.

First-line fertility treatments, unless a woman or her partner has specific medical conditions, should focus on diet, lifestyle, weight management, and supplementation to address nutrient deficiency.

This is especially true for PCOS women because PCOS improves dramatically with lifestyle interventions.

Study after study has shown that a high-nutrient diet enhances fertility in women with PCOS. Women who are overweight substantially increase fertility by losing 5% to 10% of their body weight. Meal-timing, exercise, and stress reduction all improve metabolic health and increase fertility.

And certain supplements and vitamins can regulate ovulation and improve egg quality, thereby increasing fertility.

If you have PCOS and you want to get pregnant, you should try lifestyle modifications first.

And you need to start these strategies *before* you get pregnant. This is key. Good health is foundational to a successful pregnancy, especially a successful PCOS pregnancy. That means getting healthy first.

I believe that all women, and PCOS women in particular, should take at least three months to get their health in order before attempting to get pregnant.

That's the approach that this book takes.

For 12 weeks, focus on your health. Get your blood sugar and insulin resistance under control. Lose weight. Restore your gut and vaginal microbiomes. Adopt a high-nutrient, high-fiber diet and a moderate exercise program. Remove hormone-disrupting chemicals from your food and environment. Stabilize your circadian rhythm. Monitor your ovulation patterns, and do everything you can to start ovulating if you aren't right now.

And for these 12 weeks, use a natural form of birth control such as condoms or fertility awareness. Do not use birth control pills, an intrauterine device (IUD), or any other hormonal birth control such as a ring or implant. For 12 weeks, while you focus on optimizing your health, pay attention to your natural menstrual cycle, but do not get pregnant.

If you are yearning for a bright-eyed baby, you may find this advice tough to swallow. But it's really important. Invest 12 weeks in laying the groundwork for a safe, successful pregnancy.

Some parts of this fertility protocol, such as fasting, are excellent for optimizing your health but are not safe to do while pregnant. Some herbs are great for getting ovulation up and running but are not safe to use while pregnant.

Dedicate the next 12 weeks to you and your health. By the end of these three months, you'll be healthier, your eggs will be healthier, and you'll have a solid understanding of your ovulation cycle. After 12 weeks, you will be ready to try to get pregnant.

What is the PCOS SOS Fertility Fast Track?

This book is the daughter of my bestselling book PCOS SOS.

PCOS SOS *Fertility Fast Track* turns over 350 pages of science, tips, and advice into a 12-week plan that guides you to optimal health and fertility, complete with shopping lists, check lists, menu ideas, and schedules.

If you have PCOS, you know achieving optimal health is a challenge. It takes time, dedication, consistency, and resolve. No matter where you are in your PCOS journey, you can reclaim your health and fertility. I've helped many women like you do so. It won't be easy (change never is), but you can do this! This guide will make it as easy as possible.

Throughout this book, I try my best to walk the line between giving you enough information to remind you why each lifestyle change enhances health and fertility without providing so much information that I turn this book into a textbook. This is meant to be a fast track afterall and that means concise.

At any point, if you want a more detailed explanation, please refer to PCOS SOS. Like a good mother, she knows everything!

My promise to you

I wish I could promise that if you follow this 12-week protocol, you will get pregnant and you will carry your baby to term. No one can promise you that. If your PCOS is exceptionally severe, you may need longer than three months to restore your health and fertility. You may have additional fertility issues beyond PCOS. Your partner may have fertility complications.

No matter what, even if you follow this protocol to a T, you will still have PCOS. If you have PCOS now, you will have it forever. PCOS is a natural female variant, not a disease. It only acts like a disease because our western lifestyles and diets are so dysfunctional.

PCOS used to be a mild condition. It's inherited, which means that you likely got it from your mother, who got it from her mother, who got it from hers. Your ancestral foremothers had PCOS but were fertile. They had the more mild, historical version of PCOS. Not the crazy, debilitating version that is so common today.

The PCOS SOS *Fertility Fast Track* is designed to turn your more aggressive form of PCOS into the mild form that your foremothers had. You will still have PCOS, but it will no longer feel like a disease.

I can't promise you a baby.

What I can promise is that if you follow this protocol, you will be dramatically healthier in 12 weeks than you are today.

Your metabolism and hormonal profile will be better. Your body will have less inflammation and less insulin resistance. Your eggs will be higher quality. You will be more fertile.

You will put the odds in your favor.

If that's not enough for you to get pregnant naturally and if you do end up needing more invasive fertility treatments, your improved health will make those treatments safer and more effective.

And no matter how you ultimately end up building your family, if you follow this protocol and maintain the habits that this book establishes, you will have laid the groundwork for a lifetime of healthy PCOS mamahood, which is exactly what you and your future babies deserve.

PART ONE

Before we begin

CHAPTER 1

————

PCOS: A quick explanation of a complicated condition

Pronunciation guides

In my books, I always include medical terms and their pronunciations because I believe in patient health literacy. It's easier to research when you know the proper name for something, and it's easier to discuss a symptom with your doctor when you know you are saying its name correctly.

PCOS (PEE-see-oh-ehs) is the acronym for Polycystic Ovary Syndrome. Its name makes it sound like a disease, but it is not. Officially, it is an endocrine (EN-duh-krin) disorder, which is a hormone disorder. But really, PCOS is a natural endocrine difference.

Across all races and ethnicities worldwide, approximately 10% of women have PCOS, and these rates have been fairly consistent for ages. In fact, PCOS has been around for at least 50,000 years.[1]

It is a natural female variant. PCOS is not a disease. It's simply a hormonal difference that a subset of women are born with, and it's been this way for thousands of years.

Your grandmothers and great-great-great grandmothers had the historical form of PCOS, a mild condition that, in many ways, was an evolutionary advantage. Mild inflammation meant that their immune systems were always ready to fight disease. Mild sugar intolerance meant that they carried just a few extra pounds, and mild metabolic differences helped them survive famines. Mildly elevated testosterone levels helped them build muscles and made them strong. And mild infertility decreased the number of children they bore, increased the number of years between pregnancies, and, consequently, decreased their risk of dying in childbirth.

PCOS today has become disease-like because our hormonal differences make us less able to live in today's dysfunctional society. More than non-

PCOS women, we need a natural, nurturing environment to keep our PCOS in a natural, mild state.

When we eat processed foods and sit too much, when we live and work in windowless buildings away from the rhythms of the day and night, when we expose our bodies to hormone-mimicking chemicals, we get sick, really sick. Sicker than non-PCOS women. Mild inflammation becomes chronic, whole-body inflammation. Mild sugar intolerance becomes diabetes. Mild metabolic differences become obesity. Mildly elevated testosterone levels become chronic acne. And mild infertility becomes absolute infertility.

What used to be a difference is now a disorder.

PCOS symptoms

The PCOS of today affects a woman's whole body. This is a complex condition with literally dozens of symptoms.

Each woman with PCOS will have her own, unique version of this condition. But if you have PCOS, here is an A to Z list of some of the symptoms you might be experiencing:

- **Acanthosis nigricans (ah-can-THO-sis NEE-gree-cans):** patches of velvety, darkened skin, which are associated with elevated blood sugar levels.

- **Acne:** chronic skin infections on the face and back, including deep cystic (SIS-tik) acne.

- **Alopecia (ah-loe-PEE-shah):** thinning scalp hair.

- **Autoimmune disease, especially Hashimoto's Thyroiditis (haw-she-MOE-toes THY-royd-aye-tis):** immune system dysfunction that causes the body to attack itself; in the case of Hashimoto's, the body attacks the thyroid gland.

- **Cancer, especially endometrial (en-doe-MEE-hgtree-all) cancer:** disease marked by abnormal cell growth that can spread and become life-threatening; there are hundreds of types of cancers, each of which is caused by a complex interaction of multiple risk factors.

- **Cardiovascular disease:** heart disease; narrowing of the blood vessels caused by inflammation and the buildup of plaque; can lead to heart attack and stroke.

- **Diabetes (dy-ah-BEE-teez):** the inability of the body to regulate the amount of sugar in the blood.

- **Eating disorders, specifically binge-eating disorder and bulimia (bull-EE-me-ah) nervosa:** behavior disorders marked by over-eating; they are classified as mood disorders, and binge-eating and bulimia often have a hormonal imbalance component.

- **Fatty liver disease:** accumulation of fatty tissue in the liver that causes metabolic dysfunction and liver scarring, which can lead to liver failure.

- **Gastroesophageal Reflux (GERD):** irritation in the esophagus caused by stomach acid backwash; also called heartburn or acid indigestion.

- **Gum disease, specifically gingivitis (jin-juh-VAHY-tis) and periodontal (per-ee-uh-DON-tl) disease:** infection and inflammation of the gums around the teeth.

- **Hirsutism (HER-soo-tizm):** dark hair growth on a woman's face, abdomen, legs, chest, and back.

- **Hypertension:** high blood pressure.

- **Infertility and subfertility:** difficulty becoming pregnant or maintaining a pregnancy up to a live birth delivery.

- **Insomnia (in-SOM-nee-ah):** difficulty falling or staying asleep.

- **Irritable bowel syndrome (IBS):** any combination of frequent abdominal pain, bloating, gas, diarrhea, and constipation.

- **Menstrual irregularity or absence:** infrequent, irregular, or absent periods.

- **Miscarriage:** unintended pregnancy loss.

- **Mood disorders, specifically anxiety and depression:** mental health conditions where a person's emotions are too strong (too happy, too sad, or too worried) for the situation they are in.

- **Obesity:** an unhealthy amount of body fat.

- **Pregnancy complications:**
    - **Preeclampsia (pree-i-KLAMP-see-uh):** high blood pressure accompanied by swelling in hands and feet and organ damage, indicated by protein in urine.
    - **Gestational (jeh-STAY-shun-all) diabetes:** pregnancy-onset diabetes.
    - **Macrosomia (mack-roh-SOHM-ee-ah):** very large baby, which increases the risk of delivery complications for mother and baby and is an independent risk for long term metabolic disorders for the baby.
    - **Preterm delivery:** birth before 37 weeks, associated with poorer infant health outcomes.

- **Skin tags:** little nubs of excess skin.

- **Sleep apnea (AP-nee-ah):** when a person momentarily stops breathing while asleep; may or may not be accompanied by snoring.

- **Stroke:** a brain injury caused by a blood vessel that either bursts or becomes blocked.

- **Thrombophilia (thrahm-bo-FILL-ee-ah):** a blood coagulation disorder that increases a person's risk of developing blood clots; this disorder is associated with pregnancy complications and recurrent pregnancy loss.

This expansive, whole-body-encompassing list of symptoms is the primary reason I so strongly dislike the name, Polycystic Ovary Syndrome. A condition that impacts every organ and system in the female body is reduced to the appearance of a woman's ovaries.

A complex endocrine disorder

PCOS is not an ovary disorder. It is an endocrine disorder that develops from a normal endocrine difference.

Your endocrine system is your body's hormonal messenger system. It includes the collection of glands that make hormones, chemical messengers that travel throughout your body and orchestrate the behaviors of your organs and systems, all the way down to the cellular level. The endocrine system includes the receptors for hormones that are located on virtually every cell in your body and the enzymes that control the release and degradation of those hormones.

An endocrine disorder is any ailment that involves the over- or under-production of hormones or any part of the transport, reception, and elimination of hormones.

PCOS is an endocrine disorder that is characterized by high levels of androgen hormones, usually testosterone (one of the key "male" hormones). This is accompanied by slightly lower levels of estrogen (your "female" hormone) that don't rise and fall properly throughout the menstrual cycle.

In a non-PCOS woman, estrogen levels vary considerably throughout ovulation and menstruation in a repeating monthly rhythm, but in PCOS women, estrogen levels remain much more stable and fairly low, which is one of the primary contributing factors to irregular or absent menstruation.

Estrogen dominance

Sometimes, people talk about PCOS as an "estrogen dominance" condition. I really dislike this term. In PCOS, the problem isn't that you have too much estrogen; it's that your estrogen never properly spikes to trigger ovulation.

Levels of estradiol (es-truh-DIE-all), the primary estrogen in reproductive-aged women, vary dramatically throughout the menstrual cycle, ranging from 15 to 350 pg/mL, or higher. For ovulation to occur, estradiol must spike to above 300 pg/ML, and at the end of a menstrual cycle, levels may fall as low as 15 pg/mL. In contrast, women with PCOS often have estradiol levels that are chronically between 60 and 90 pg/mL, which is in the lower third of the full estrogen range.

The term "estrogen dominance" refers to relatively low levels of progesterone (pro-JEH-steh-rohn), another sex hormone, seen in PCOS women. Women with PCOS have too much estradiol relative to progesterone. It's not that they have high estrogen; it's that compared to their estrogen levels, they have a relative progesterone deficiency.[2]

The solution is not to drive down estrogen. It's to normalize the estrogen cycle, which, in turn, normalizes progesterone as well as all of the other hormones involved in ovulation and menstruation.

In women, estrogen is what I call the "Master Hormone." There are estrogen receptors on virtually every cell in every organ in your body. You have estrogen receptors in your uterus and vagina, in your bladder, on your immune cells, throughout your digestive tract, in your heart, lungs, skin, and throughout your brain. Every part of your body has evolved to need rhythmically cycling estrogen to function optimally.

Because many of the other hormones in your body are tied to estrogen, women with PCOS have abnormal levels of testosterone, progesterone, luteinizing hormone (LH), follicular stimulating hormone (FSH), melatonin, cortisol, and anti-Müllerian hormone (AMH). These hormones regulate critical functions throughout your body, including reproduction, mood, hunger, sleep, and your immune system.

A quick hormone primer

Hormones are messenger molecules. Cells that respond to specific hormones contain specific receptors for those hormones. You can think of hormones as keys and receptors as locks. Each type of hormone can only fit into receptors designed for that hormone. When a hormone fits into its appropriate receptor on a cell, it unlocks a behavior in that cell, and in this way, hormones control all of the organs and systems in your body.

There are approximately 50 unique hormones in the human body. These are a few you should know about:

* **Anti-Müllerian hormone (AMH):** Every woman of reproductive age has a number of semi-developed, resting egg follicles in her ovaries. These follicles secrete a small, steady amount of AMH. Consequently, AMH can be a marker for how many high quality eggs a woman has. High

AMH usually indicates good ovarian reserve. Unfortunately, PCOS women tend to have such a high number of partially developed follicles that we often have abnormally high AMH, and when AMH gets too high, it blocks ovulation.

- **Cortisol (CORE-tuh-sall):** This is your primary stress hormone. Cortisol also plays a role in hunger, metabolism, mood, and your sleep-wake cycle. Ideally, cortisol is high in the morning to wake you up and encourage you to eat breakfast, and then it slowly drops throughout the day so you can fall asleep and fast all night. Women with PCOS overproduce cortisol and we don't metabolize it correctly. We also have an abnormal 24-hour cortisol cycle. This makes us prone to over-eating, weight gain, mood problems, and sleep disorders.[3,4]

- **Estrogen:** Estrogen is the primary female sex hormone and is also the Master Homone in women's bodies. It controls reproduction, immune function, energy production, and the circadian rhythm. Because almost every cell in your body has estrogen receptors, estrogen supports the function of every organ in your body. There are four types:

  - **Estrone (E1):** The primary estrogen in post-menopausal older women.

  - **Estradiol (E2):** The primary estrogen in women of reproductive age, and the most potent estrogen. In normally menstruating women, levels of estradiol elevate dramatically to trigger ovulation and then plummet during menstruation. In women with PCOS, estradiol levels often remain low and relatively stable.

- **Estriol (E3):** An estrogen that plays a critical role in pregnancy.

- **Estetrol (E4):** An estrogen produced by both male and female fetuses during pregnancy.

Improperly cycling estradiol is one of the foundational causes of PCOS hormonal imbalances.

- **Follicular stimulating hormone (FSH):** FSH helps regulate the production of estradiol, and in ovulation, FSH is required for an ovarian follicle to mature and release its egg. In women with PCOS, FSH is usually low to normal. Low FSH results in suboptimal estradiol production and can prevent an egg follicle from maturing, which prevents ovulation.

- **Insulin (IN-suh-lin):** Released by the pancreas, insulin is a sugar and fat-regulating hormone. When blood sugar increases, insulin causes cells to absorb sugar (technically, insulin tells a cell to transport glucose across its cell membrane and into the cell) for cell metabolism. "Insulin sensitivity" describes how sensitive cells are to insulin. High insulin sensitivity means that cells need only a little insulin to induce sugar absorption. Poor insulin sensitivity, also called "insulin resistance," occurs when cells begin to ignore insulin and, consequently, much more insulin is required to trigger cell sugar absorption. In general, insulin sensitivity is good; insulin resistance is bad and leads to diabetes.

High insulin levels also cause increased fat production and storage, specifically as visceral, or belly, fat. Virtually all PCOS women have high insulin levels and are insulin resistant, and even normal weight and thin women with PCOS have higher amounts of visceral fat compared with same-weight non-PCOS women.

- **Luteinizing hormone (LH):** Like FSH, LH supports the developing egg follicle. In the early days of the menstrual cycle, a woman produces similar amounts of LH and FSH, but when ovulation approaches, estrogen spikes and triggers a similar, dramatic spike in LH, which causes the egg to release. In PCOS women, LH is constantly elevated. Without a proper estrogen spike, LH can't spike so it just stays abnormally high. It is common for PCOS women to have an LH to FSH ratio greater than 2:1, which means that a woman is producing more than twice as much LH as FSH. Unfortunately, LH has a second job—it encourages your body to produce more testosterone, which is actually a precursor of estrogen. High LH leads to high testosterone production, and without adequate FSH, this testosterone can't be converted into estrogen. So high LH contributes to hyperandrogenism.

- **Melatonin (mell-uh-TONE-in):** This is your sleep hormone. It is typically low throughout the day and begins to rise in the late evening. In addition to inducing sleep, melatonin is a powerful antioxidant that protects a woman's eggs from oxidative damage. Women with PCOS have dysfunctional melatonin pathways—high levels of melatonin but poor melatonin function, including poor sleep and high levels of oxidative damage, especially in the ovaries. Melatonin supplements often correct these problems.[5,6]

- **Progesterone:** After ovulation, the empty egg follicle, called a corpus luteum, releases progesterone. This hormone causes the uterine lining to thicken to accept a fertilized egg, called a zygote (ZY-gote). If the zygote implants, it immediately forms a placenta, which begins secreting progesterone and maintains the uterine lining. The corpus luteum lasts for about two weeks and then shrinks. Without a fertilized egg and placenta, progesterone drops, the uterine lining sheds, and menstruation begins. Women with PCOS often have low progesterone, which impedes implantation.

- **Testosterone (tess-TOSS-ter-own):** Testosterone is the primary androgen, or male hormone, in both men and women. (Your body has about 10% of the testosterone that a man's body has.) Proper female testosterone levels support sexual and mental health and the growth of strong bones and muscles. PCOS women, compared to non-PCOS women, have mildly elevated levels of testosterone or other androgens such as androstenedione or dehydroepiandrosterone sulfate (DHEA-S). This causes acne, hirsutism, and alopecia. Although initially controversial, it now seems that elevated androgens also cause inflammation, insulin resistance, and infertility. The more testosterone you have, the more severe your PCOS symptoms are.

Consequently, when estrogen doesn't do what it is supposed to do, every organ and system in your body suffers. All of the foundational rhythms in your body—digestion, hunger, metabolism, sleep, healing, and detoxification, to name a few—get off rhythm and out of sync with each other. The end result is that every part of your body needs to work harder to do its job and keep you alive.

This means that every organ in your body is under some degree of stress. Low-grade, chronic stress causes chronic, systemic inflammation.

Inflammation damages metabolism, which is the management of energy in your body. Metabolism is an intricate process that coordinates all of your organs in perfect synchronicity, guided by your body's 24-hour daily rhythms, which we call your circadian rhythm. In addition to your liver, pancreas, your entire digestive tract, and all of the fat cells in your body, metabolism involves your bones, muscles, immune system, and of course, brain.

At its most basic level, metabolism can be reduced to the consumption, creation, and storage of glucose (sugar) and lipids (fats), which are your body's main sources of energy. Most of the time, your body runs on sugar. Blood sugar is regulated by the hormone insulin, and a key marker of metabolic dysfunction is insulin resistance. Any time your body runs out of sugar due to exercise, fasting, or a low-carb diet, you must switch to fat metabolism, a complex process that involves the pancreas, liver, brain, kidneys, and fat cells. Maintaining energy balance in the body is a massive physiological undertaking that relies on precise hormonal coordination.

This delicate metabolic synchronization is off-the-beat in PCOS women. Our bodies love to stay in sugar-burning, fat-storage mode. We typically have a hard time switching from sugar metabolism to fat metabolism. This leads to chronic hunger and weight-gain.

The exact means by which low, a-rhythmic estrogen causes all of the symptoms found across PCOS women is complex and poorly understood. In addition to all of the processes I've described, there are additional hormones from adipose (fat) tissue and the cells that line your intestines that are produced off-rhythm and at improper levels. There are growth hormones and immune cells that contribute to chronic inflammation.

Our bodies seem to be resistant to a wide range of hormones beyond insulin.

In PCOS SOS, I explain in depth how poor aromatization (the conversion of testosterone to estrogen) is the root cause of PCOS and how this cascades into whole-body dysfunction. Studies on the etiology of PCOS are ongoing and our understanding is constantly evolving.

PCOS is an extremely complex condition that truly involves every organ, hormone, and cell in your body. Fortunately, you don't need to understand the complete underlying pathology because, at the end of the day, everyone agrees that there are three foundational challenges in a PCOS woman's body:

1. Widespread hormonal imbalance
2. Chronic inflammation
3. Insulin resistance

These three conditions are the underlying causes of the myriad PCOS symptoms that you are suffering from. Treat them and all of the other PCOS dysfunctions heal, including infertility.

It's all about inflammation and insulin resistance

Directly controlling hormones is difficult, especially if you don't want a whole slew of side effects. And the PCOS hormonal therapies available today, such as birth control pills and spironolactone (spy-roh-noh-LAK-tone), aren't safe for pregnancy anyway.

Some doctors prescribe metformin, an insulin sensitizer, to non-diabetic PCOS women. Metformin is an endocrine disruptor and there is evidence that it inflicts long-term metabolic harm on fetuses. I do not recommend metformin during pregnancy.

Estrogen replacement

I deeply, truly believe that in the future, rhythmic, bioidentical estrogen therapy *will* be the key to reversing all of the symptoms of PCOS in non-pregnant women resistant to lifestyle change and supplementation. But we desperately need studies to prove that it works and that it is safe, and we need to evaluate dosing levels. To have studies, we have to have funding. And right now, the funding isn't there. I actively work with the non-profit PCOS Challenge to change that!

The most effective PCOS treatments focus on reducing inflammation and improving insulin resistance. Incredibly, when we get inflammation and insulin resistance under control, hormones almost always normalize, at least to a historical PCOS level where healthy fertility and metabolism are restored.

As I discuss in PCOS SOS, the most effective lifestyle modifications you can adopt to lower inflammation and insulin resistance are:

1. Establish a strong circadian rhythm, using light and darkness, sleep, and time-restricted eating.
2. Nurture a healthy gut microbiome with diet and exercise.
3. Avoid endocrine disruptors.

These are the strategies that you will use in this Fertility Fast Track, along with some additional strategies to optimize your detoxification pathways, restore your vaginal microbiome, and track ovulation.

Getting your PCOS diagnosis

Before we get too far, I want to emphasize how important it is to get a true PCOS diagnosis from a doctor. PCOS is technically a "syndrome" which means it is diagnosed when a woman has specific symptoms *and* other possible diagnoses have been ruled out.

Your doctor will take your medical history, order blood tests, and possibly recommend a transvaginal ultrasound.

There are a couple of different competing diagnosis criteria for PCOS. The definition that I find most useful is the one developed by the Androgen Excess and PCOS Society (AE-PCOS). This definition was recently reaffirmed at an international symposium hosted by the Centre for Research Excellence in Polycystic Ovary Syndrome (CRE PCOS) in 2018. According to the AE-PCOS Society and the CRE PCOS, a woman has PCOS if she has:

1. **Hyperandrogenism (hy-per-AN-dro-jen-izm):** an above average level of androgens, male sex hormones such as testosterone. This is a *required* symptom. Hyperandrogenism can be documented through a blood test or by observing symptoms of elevated androgen levels, such as acne, dark hair in places where normally only men get it (face, chest, back), and thinning hair on the scalp.

Additionally, for a PCOS diagnosis, a woman must have one or both of the following symptoms:

2. **Irregular or absent menstruation (in women of reproductive age):** an irregular cycle is anything less frequent than once every 35 days, anything more frequent than every 21 days, a cycle that varies in length by more than a few days, or a cycle where bleeding lasts longer than 7 days.

3. **Polycystic ovaries, as seen on an ultrasound.**

Polycystic ovaries

What *are* polycystic ovaries? This isn't as scary as it sounds. Due to hormonal imbalances, the ovaries contain many enlarged follicles.

All women's ovaries are full of follicles, tiny fluid-filled sacs that each contain a single, immature egg. When ovulation occurs properly, one follicle grows and develops each month until the egg bursts from the follicle (ovulation!) and travels down the fallopian tube into the uterus. If it is not fertilized by sperm, the egg disintegrates or leaves the body along with the lining of the uterus (menstruation!).

At the start of a normal menstrual cycle, many follicles begin to develop, but only one is recruited to fully develop and release its egg. When that follicle is chosen, the other follicles regress, or shrivel up. In a healthy ovary, you may see several tiny follicles or one larger, more mature follicle.

In women with PCOS, no specific follicle gets recruited to be the one to ovulate, and so a large number of developing follicles continue to exist. These follicles are sometimes described as a "string of pearls" because they form along the outer rim of the ovary.

These cysts are not dangerous. But when no single egg fully matures and bursts from its sack, ovulation does not occur. And then a woman doesn't get her period regularly. Lack of regular ovulation is a major cause of the infertility suffered by so many women with PCOS.

Polycystic ovaries are diagnosed through a transvaginal ultrasound and are evidence of the broken ovulation process. They don't cause PCOS. They are a symptom of PCOS.

PCOS is a diagnosis of exclusion. There are other conditions, really serious conditions, that can look like PCOS. Only a doctor can rule out endocrine tumors, Cushing's Syndrome, congenital and acquired adrenal hyperplasia, and other endocrine disorders.

If you are experiencing PCOS symptoms but don't have a diagnosis from a doctor, please make an appointment right away. If your doctor doesn't take your symptoms seriously or simply recommends pharmaceuticals (birth control pills, metformin, or Clomid) find a new doctor. A proper diagnosis along with support for lifestyle interventions is critical.

CHAPTER 2

The Fertility Fast
Track protocol

Over the next 12 weeks, I will guide you through a rigorous get-healthy-and-fertile protocol. Many of the recommendations come from my previous book, PCOS SOS, but some of them are new and specifically aimed at enhancing fertility.

All of these therapies focus on food, supplements, and lifestyle changes.

Our culture conditions us to think of pharmaceuticals as powerful medicine and lifestyle choices, such as diet and sleep, as nice-to-have wellness routines. This is wrong. Food is medicine. Sleep is medicine. Sunlight and darkness are medicine. Exercise is medicine. Supplements are medicine. Numerous studies show that healthy choices change the way our cells functions and our genes express themselves.

The strategies in this book focus on three powerful change areas—circadian rhythm, microbiomes, and exposure to endocrine disruptors—that dramatically improve PCOS symptoms and enhance your fertility.

Circadian rhythm

Your circadian rhythm is your body's daily 24-hour cycle. Every hormone and organ system in your body has a natural 24-hour rhythm. Every one of your cells has specific genes, called clock genes, that respond to hormonal signals and drive these daily cycles.

Estrogen is intricately involved in the maintenance of healthy circadian rhythms. In the female body, estrogen modulates sleep, metabolism, digestion, and, of course, reproduction. The chronically low, a-rhythmic estrogen associated with PCOS weakens your body's circadian rhythms, causing hormonal imbalances and systemic inflammation.[1]

Circadian rhythm disruption aggravates all of your PCOS symptoms. It is also independently linked to lowered fertility. With or without PCOS, women who work at night, what we call shift work, are less fertile. Women with sleep problems are less fertile. Even women who routinely skip breakfast are less fertile. Rhythms matter.[2,3]

We women are rhythmic creatures, and our circadian rhythms are foundational to whole body and reproductive health. Repairing these rhythms is critical to repairing your fertility.

Your circadian rhythm is primarily driven by the sun. In the morning, sunlight enters your eyes and entrains your master clock, or your suprachiasmatic nucleus, a part of your brain that sends circadian signals to all of the other cells in your body.

Many of the strategies in this book will focus on creating a powerful light-to-dark daily pattern that will set your body's clocks.

Sleep is another essential piece of the day-night, 24-hour pattern. So we will make sure you get sufficient, highly restorative sleep every night.

The clocks in your digestive tract are actually set by your gut microbiome, not your brain, and they need to be perfectly synced to the other clocks in your body. The digestive circadian rhythm is cued by eating and fasting. Your body interprets eating as daytime and fasting as nighttime, so we will use a technique called "time-restricted eating" to establish a robust and healthy digestive circadian rhythm that corresponds to your light-dark, wake-sleep circadian rhythms.

Microbiomes

The human body evolved to be dependent on the microbes that cover the skin and populate the digestive tract, mouth, vagina, and other organs.

Your gut microbiome is the largest microbe population in your body.

It contributes to circadian rhythm by setting the cellular clocks throughout your digestive tract. These clocks play a critical role in metabolism, and by regulating your liver function, they modulate insulin sensitivity.

Additionally, these gut microbes communicate directly with your immune system so a healthy microbiome lowers inflammation. And these microbes are hormonally active, producing and responding to human hormones and neurotransmitters. There is even a special part of the gut microbiome, called the estrobolome, that controls the breakdown and conservation of your naturally occurring estrogen. A healthy estrobolome recycles the estrogen your body produces in a precise way to naturally increase your estrogen levels.

Your gut microbiome is nurtured primarily by food. The microbes in your intestines thrive when you eat a plant-heavy, high-fiber, minimally processed diet. For reasons that we are only starting to understand, your gut microbiome also needs you to exercise regularly.

Consequently, the plan in this book will show you how to eat a microbiome-healthy diet and start a moderate exercise program.

We will also focus on eliminating the biggest microbiome killers—antibiotics, alcohol, sugar, excessive fat, and synthetic food additives.

Your gut microbiome is your body's biggest microbiome, but when it comes to fertility, there are two additional microbiomes that we need to take care of.

In your mouth, your oral microbiome is critical for digesting and absorbing nutrients. It plays an essential role in your body's creation of a compound called nitric oxide (NIGH-trik OX-ide), which protects your heart and blood vessels. In pregnancy, dental diseases caused by pathogenic bacteria significantly increase the risk of preeclampsia and preterm birth.[4]

Your vagina is home to its own unique microbiome which is equally critical for an uncomplicated pregnancy. Vaginal infections increase rates of miscarriage, preterm birth, low birth weight, and labor and delivery complications. Your vaginal microbiome is the first microbiome to colonize your baby, so you want it to be healthy.[5,6]

Over the next 12 weeks, you will nurture stable, diverse, and healthy microbiomes in your gut, mouth, and vagina.

Endocrine disruptors

Our modern world is full of synthetic chemicals that interact with our endocrine system and change the way our hormones function. They are found in plastics, nonstick cookware, processed foods, cleaning and beauty products, sunscreen, pesticides, and drinking water.

PCOS women tend to have higher blood levels of a wide range of industrial endocrine-disrupting chemicals, and higher levels of chemicals correspond to more severe PCOS symptoms. Endocrine disruptors are also independently tied to infertility and adverse pregnancy outcomes.[7,8]

On top of that, in pregnant women, many of these chemicals can cross the placenta and harm the fetus. These chemicals change the baby's genetic programming and predispose her to chronic conditions such as diabetes and heart disease later in life. In fact, fetal exposure to bisphenol A (BPA) and phthalates, two common endocrine disruptors, has actually been linked to the development of PCOS.[9,10]

Although it is impossible to completely avoid these chemicals, it is completely possible to dramatically lower your exposure.

Over the next 12 weeks, I'll show you how to remove these chemicals from your diet, personal products, and home.

Additional fertility-enhancing strategies

Female fertility is complex and responds robustly to a wide range of lifestyle factors and environmental cues that indicate whether or not right now is a safe time to have a baby. The female body is highly motivated to increase fertility in times of abundance and decrease fertility in times of conflict and scarcity. As much as your body wants to make a baby, it also wants to protect you.

Nutrition (more than calories) is a key indicator of food abundance and social stability, so female fertility is tied to nutrition. Your ovaries require significant micronutrients, trace elements, and antioxidants obtained through diet to function properly. Without a nutrient-rich diet, your ovaries atrophy (shrink) and become damaged by molecules called free radicals, a process known as oxidative stress. This plan optimizes your diet to provide you with a constant stream of high-quality and varied nutrients.[11]

Emotional wellbeing also affects fertility. Women who have high levels of alpha-amylase, a marker for chronic emotional stress, are more than

50% more likely to experience infertility than women with normal alpha-amylase levels. Stress changes a variety of hormone levels, which disrupts signaling needed for successful ovulation and implantation. Stress (and infertility can be immensely stressful) is also really bad for you as a woman and as a human being. I will teach you some simple techniques to manage stress.[12,13]

Although knowledge itself doesn't increase fertility, it helps you make the most of the fertility you have, and it helps you make informed decisions about what steps to take throughout your fertility journey. When you make changes in your lifestyle, you may find it hard to know if these changes are having a positive impact. Every week, you will monitor several excellent markers for inflammation and metabolic health: your weight, BMI, waist circumference, and blood pressure. You will also monitor your ovulation using an ovulation tracker. Reasonably regular ovulation is a sign that your hormones are cycling normally. Throughout this program, you will monitor health markers so you have insight into what is happening within your body.

Let's talk about health

A major goal of this fast track program is to help you get healthier. What does that mean? I think of health as the ability to physically and emotionally do the things in life that are important to you.

You get to decide what your own definition of health is. What activities make you happy? Do you like to travel, hike, camp, swim, or play sports? Do you need to lift heavy items or stand on your feet for long stretches? Do you want to stay calm in the face of an emergency? Do you require the emotional reserves to be a caregiver? Do you hope to have a baby?

Health isn't a number; it's a capacity to live a rewarding life as you define it. And it's the capacity to maintain that life for as long into the future as possible.

Even though there isn't a single portrait of health, we do know that certain health factors increase or decrease your risk for long-term illnesses and conditions that could ultimately lower your quality of life.

As a doctor, I try very hard to walk the line between honoring all of my patients wherever they are in their health journeys while also being honest about risk factors that I see in their blood work, weight, and lifestyle. My goal is always to provide information and a path, without judgment.

You are not your health numbers. But your numbers do mean something.

This is especially true when it comes to pregnancy. Excess weight, insulin resistance, and high blood pressure, testosterone, and blood levels of endocrine disruptors such as BPA, mercury, and lead identify risks to your health, fertility, and the well-being of your future babies.

For a healthy pregnancy and a healthy baby, we are going to need to look at your health numbers.

Let's talk about weight

Weight is probably the hardest number to talk about because, more than any other health metric, weight is not just a number.

Most women with PCOS are overweight. Our dysfunctional metabolism, insulin resistance, and chronic inflammation mean that our bodies are always in fat storage mode, and when we store fat, we are more likely to store it in our bellies (visceral fat) than in our thighs and butts. This is why so many PCOS women develop the infamous "apple shape," which is associated with an increased risk of heart disease, and not the much less dangerous "pear shape."

We all know that our extra weight isn't good for us. But I'm sure you've also noticed that if you have PCOS and are overweight, losing weight with PCOS is *hard*! Our bodies are metabolically thrifty. We naturally conserve energy and store this energy as fat. Historically, this meant that our foremothers were really good at surviving famines. Sadly, this is not a trait that is all that useful anymore.

So, we PCOS women tend to gain weight. Once we gain it, we tend to keep it. And we live in a society that can be really mean to any woman who isn't perfectly skinny.

I absolutely do not want to make you feel guilty about your body. Your body is a gift from every powerful woman who came before you, and it is designed to thrive in a natural environment full of daily rhythms, exercise, and natural foods. Your body isn't defective, but your environment is.

Being overweight is a sign that your body is struggling to live in today's toxic and unnatural world. This plan will help you heal your body by showing you how to change your environment to make it more similar to the environments that allowed our foremothers to thrive.

As a doctor, I want to say this about weight, and in particular about weight, PCOS, and pregnancy: You do not have to be skinny to be healthy.

But, if you are overweight, you will improve your fertility and make your pregnancy safer by losing weight. Losing weight is also a visible signal that you are lowering inflammation and improving insulin resistance.

This plan will show you how to lose weight in a way that is healthy and sustainable. You will likely need to change what you eat and when you eat, but I do not advocate calorie-restrictive dieting. You don't need to count calories, limit calories, or even know what a calorie is.

Short-term fasting, on the other hand, is a fabulous way to reset your metabolism, circadian rhythm, and gut microbiome, so I will ask you to do three rounds of a Fasting Mimicking Diet (more on that later). During the first few days of each Fasting Mimicking Diet, you may feel food-deprived. But, aside from when you are actively fasting, I will never ask you to go hungry.

Remember, I define health as the capacity to live a full and rewarding life. Constant hunger is not conducive to happiness. Constant hunger isn't healthy.

Lean PCOS women

If you are one of the approximately 20% of PCOS women who are not overweight, don't feel left out. This plan will help you, too.

For overweight women, weight loss is a sign of an improving metabolism. If you are already at a healthy weight, you will get healthier on this program without losing much, if any, weight, and maintaining your weight should get easier.

f you are a lean PCOS woman with fertility challenges, you are almost certainly insulin resistant. The supplements, lifestyle modifications, and dietary changes in this book will help.

So long as your body mass index (BMI) is above 18, you should follow this plan exactly as it is, including the fasts.

If your BMI is below 20, you should discuss with your doctor whether you should actually gain a little weight to maximize your fertility.

If your BMI is below 18, you should definitely gain some weight. Follow this Fertility Fast Track program, but do not participate in the Fasting Mimicking Diets.

Let's talk about true fertility

Fertility is not just about getting pregnant. That's only the first step. True fertility also encompasses the ability to have a healthy, full-term pregnancy, birth, and baby.

One of the biggest causes of infertility among PCOS women is lack of ovulation. So throughout these 12 weeks, you will monitor your ovulation. By the end of the program, you will know if you are ovulating and how often. If you follow the program and you are still not ovulating, you will know that, too.

But lack of ovulation is only part of the story. PCOS significantly increases your risk of miscarriage. Hormonal imbalances and low egg quality both play a role. PCOS decreases the health of your eggs, so I will recommend supplements that will improve your egg quality.

PCOS makes your whole body less resilient under stress. And once you get pregnant, your body will be under immense stress. This program optimizes your metabolic health so your body is able to grow a baby without getting dangerously sick or going into labor too soon.

Following this program will give you the best chance possible of having a successful pregnancy and a healthy baby. This is what I think of as true fertility.

Male (or partner) health and fertility

If your partner is a man, he needs to be healthy, too. A healthy man produces healthy sperm.

In nearly half of all couples struggling with infertility, male infertility or subfertility plays a role. Because we already know that you have fertility challenges due to PCOS, it is exceptionally important to maximize the fertility of your partner.

I am so thrilled that my friend and colleague, Professor Kelton Tremellen, has included in the back of this book a mini-guide specifically for male partners about optimizing male fertility (see page 293). Please encourage your partner to read this important section.

Not surprisingly, although men and women have some unique considerations, in general, what's good for female fertility is good for male fertility, and vice versa.

Consequently, I strongly recommend that you and your partner embark on this fertility protocol together. Have your partner follow Dr. Tremellen's advice regarding supplements and unique male fertility needs. All of my additional Fertility Fast Track lifestyle components—the diet, fasting, sleep regimen, exercise, and clean living—are universally healthy recommendations for women and men.

If you and your partner both follow the Fertility Fast Track program, you will increase your chances of successfully following it, and you will get healthier and more fertile together. Having a baby is a joint endeavor, and that starts now, before the baby is even conceived.

Let's talk about money

In the United States, there are two tiers of products—normal every-person products full of untested, minimally-regulated chemicals and high-quality, safe, natural products that are predominantly priced and marketed for economically well-off people.

It is beyond the scope of this book to argue why every person, regardless of their bank account, should have access to safe food, water, and personal care products.

But as a doctor, I have to be honest about what products and choices are best for your health and the health of your family. Whenever possible, I will show you the most cost-effective approach to improving your PCOS. And some of the advice in this book, such as cooking at home and eating less meat, will save you money. However, some of the products I recommend, such as supplements and the Fasting Mimicking Diet, cost money. They just do.

Product recommendations

I recommend products that I trust and that my patients have been successful with. For supplements, I recommend medical-grade brands that employ rigorous testing to ensure they contain exactly what they advertise and are free from contaminants. For the Fasting Mimicking Diet, ProLon is the only product on the market. In the case of home products, apps, and other items, I share what I use and enjoy.

In all cases, I don't private label my products because I don't want to have that kind of conflict of interest. I want you to know what you are buying and to have a choice in the products you purchase.

I do work with some companies as a medical advisor and lecturer. Please see page 339 for a complete disclosure of my business affiliations.

Study after study shows that healthy lifestyle choices lower your risk of heart disease, stroke, cancer, diabetes, and autoimmune disease.

Treating chronic illnesses is expensive. And infertility treatments can be extremely expensive.

In the short term, the choices and products in this book may seem pricey, but they will save you money in lower future healthcare costs.

I firmly believe that investing money in organic foods and products and investing time in exercise and self care are financially smart choices.

Obviously, every person has to live within their financial reality. That's just life. But we should all do the best we can.

Let's talk about real life

The PCOS SOS Fertility Fast Track is a rigorous program. It is designed to take you from wherever you are in your PCOS journey to a place of physical, emotional, and reproductive wellness. The more rigidly you follow the protocol, the better the results you'll see. It's trite, but you'll get out what you put in.

That being said, I want to give you permission to sometimes fail.

You are a human being. A glorious, messy, complicated, imperfect human being.

Do your best to follow this plan to the absolute best of your abilities. Give it your all. And when you inevitably hit a rough patch, forgive yourself and jump right back in.

If you keep going, despite the setbacks, you will get healthier. That's inevitable.

And I hope with all my heart that this program brings you to such a place of health and fertility that you become a mother—a glorious, messy, complicated, imperfect, and loving mother.

CHAPTER 3

Get ready!

*P*repping for the 12-week program will take a couple of days. I suggest giving yourself a week. Let's go over what you need to do and why. Then, use my quick-and-easy checklists to make sure you're ready to begin. Set yourself up for success!

Put "Day 1" on your calendar

The very first thing to do is pick a start date.

You'll need a few days to get ready so I recommend that you pick next Monday, or the following Monday. Research shows that people are most successful building new habits when they start on a "fresh start" date, such as the beginning of a new year, the first of the month, a birthday, or any old Monday.[1]

When picking your start date, you should keep in mind that your fasting weeks will fall on Weeks 4, 8, and 12. You won't be totally out of commission during fasting weeks, but ideally, you shouldn't have any big events such as parties, presentations, and critical business meetings. If your calendar doesn't work out perfectly and you can't fast during a scheduled fasting week, you can repeat or extend the preceding week of the Fertility Fast Track program until you have five days available for fasting. And then continue with the program as scheduled.

You need at least three weeks between rounds of fasting to recover so you should extend the program if you need to rather than swap weeks around or skip weeks.

It's totally fine to take more than 12 weeks to complete the Fertility Fast Track. Each week gets you healthier. If you have the flexibility to take more time with your PCOS preconception care, you'll be that much healthier when you do start trying to conceive.

So, with all of that in mind, pick a start date, preferably a Monday, and write it down.

I will start on _____

Get familiar with this book

Take a moment to skim through this book so you know what to expect.

The program is divided into three four-week chunks that I'm calling months, for simplicity's sake. And I assume that each of your weeks starts on a Monday.

Every week of this program follows the same pattern. The Sunday before each new week is planning day. You will read about the tasks and habits for the upcoming week, fill out a weekly menu, and go grocery shopping. You will also take all of your body measurements so you can track the impact that this program has on your metabolic health. You get all of this out of the way on Sunday so you are totally ready for Monday, the first day of the new week. On Monday, you start your new habits, implement new schedules, and make changes to your diet. Throughout the week, practice these new behaviors and figure out how to make them work for you and the realities of your life. Then on Sunday, get ready for the next week.

Each chapter lays out the weekly plan in this format:

1. An overview of the new habits and tasks for the week.
2. A meal planner so you can decide what you are going to eat for the week and build your grocery list.
3. A to-do list for any task to accomplish and items to buy.
4. A daily checklist so you can track all of the things you're supposed to be doing each day.
5. A Sunday planner for the following week.

The weeks are additive. The changes you make one week carry forward into all of the following weeks. All of the changes build on each other, so by the end of the program, your entire lifestyle will revamped to optimize your health and fertility.

The worksheets at the end of each chapter help you keep track of all your new habits so you don't have to memorize or remember anything.

Male fertility is an essential part of a couple's reproductive potential, so I have included a mini-guide to male fertility at the end of the 12-week program guide (page 293).

I've also included a workbook and appendix in the back of the book (page 303) that includes:

- Several pages to guide you through doctor appointments.
- Forms where you can chart your weight, BMI, hip and waist circumference, blood pressure, and PCOS symptoms throughout the program.
- Menu ideas to help you plan out your weekly menus.

And that's it! This book and a commitment to healing your PCOS are all you need.

Let's get started prepping for your first week.

Schedule appointments

You need to schedule preconception medical and dental appointments. Call your care providers as soon as possible. They may be busy and unable to see you right away.

Primary care physician, OB-GYN, or midwife appointment

Who will be responsible for your care throughout your trying-to-conceive months, pregnancy, and delivery? Ideally, you want to be cared for by an OB-GYN or midwife who is familiar with PCOS and is experienced with high-risk pregnancies. If you see a midwife, discuss how she will coordinate with an OB-GYN if you experience any complications during pregnancy or childbirth. Because PCOS increases your risk of complications, you need to have a plan in place if things start going wrong.

If you can, ask for a longer appointment. There is a lot of information to go over with your caregiver:

- General health work-up
- Birth control options
- Prescription review
- Substance abuse screening
- Vaginal screening
- Laboratory tests

Be sure to fill out and bring the Preconception Appointment Organizer on page 312 to your appointment. When you get your results back, if any of them are abnormal, schedule a follow-up appointment to recheck after you complete the 12-week Fertility Fast Track program.

Medical specialist appointments

If you have complicating medical conditions that are managed by specialists, make appointments with those specialists to discuss any issues that might impact your fertility or pregnancy. Additionally, review this Fertility Fast Track protocol with every doctor on your medical care team. Double check that there are no drug interaction concerns with any of the supplements recommended and make sure you are cleared to participate in the five-day Fasting Mimicking Diet. Bring the Specialist Appointment Organizer on page 320 to your appointment.

Dental appointment

Make an appointment with your dentist to assess your oral health. Get a general exam, and if you are due for any x-rays, get those done, too. If you need any dental work, schedule it for sometime within the next 12 weeks, so it's all taken care of before you start trying to get pregnant. If you need any fillings, make sure the fillings are mercury-free because amalgam (50% mercury) fillings are linked to an increased risk of perinatal death. However, for any amalgam fillings you already have, leave them alone. Removing them at this point will increase your exposure to mercury. Additionally, it is important to resolve any gum disease because gum disease is an independent risk for preterm labor and low birth weight babies.[2,3]

Male partner doctor appointment

This isn't really your task, but if you are hoping to get pregnant with a male partner, then he needs to see his doctor as well. It's common for women to blame themselves when they and their partner can't make a baby, but in 43% of couples experiencing infertility, male infertility plays a role. Your male partner should get a semen analysis and get screened for sexually transmitted infections, substance abuse, and health conditions that could affect the quality of his sperm or his ability to engage in sex. Even common health conditions, such as obesity or diabetes, lower male fertility.

Embarking on this Fertility Fast Track program with your partner will improve your chances of successfully getting pregnant together. If your partner will be participating in the five-day Fasting Mimicking Diets with you (and he should!), then he needs to get approval from his doctor. He should also review any supplements he plans to take. He may want to bring the male fertility guide on page 293 with him to his appointment as a reference.[4]

Go health accessory shopping

There are several health tools and products that will make this 12-week journey easier and you can continue to benefit from them while you are trying to conceive and throughout pregnancy. You should buy these items as soon as you can because you will start using many of them on Day 1.

- **Blood pressure cuff:** You should buy a simple upper arm cuff digital blood pressure monitor. It's okay to use a wrist cuff if you already own one. Just be aware that it may read higher than your actual blood pressure. Bring your blood pressure cuff to your next doctor's appointment to calibrate it.

- **Fasting Mimicking Diet:** The Fasting Mimicking Diet is a five-day program developed at the Longevity Institute at the University of Southern California under the directorship of Professor Valter Longo. A start-up company, L-Nutra, was spawned from this groundbreaking research to produce a commercial version of the Fasting Mimicking Diet called ProLon (short for Promoting Longevity). The ProLon diet gives you a metabolic reboot, dramatically lowering inflammation and insulin resistance.
  Unfortunately, there are no do-it-yourself alternatives to ProLon. And there are no ways to get the incredible benefits of a five-day fast without fasting for five days.

  Each ProLon box comes with five days of food that allow you to eat while keeping your body in an extended fasting state. You will need one box for each month of the program, three total. (ProLon has a buy-three discount that helps with the cost).

Check with your doctor to make sure you are approved to fast before you purchase any ProLon kits. Also, if you have a nut allergy, you will need to skip this part of the program because ProLon includes nuts. You can purchase the ProLon diet here: ProLonfmd.com.

- **Ovulation tracker:** I highly recommend that you invest in a high-quality ovulation tracker. You need one that works for women with PCOS. We have irregular hormonal profiles and most of us have irregular cycles. You want several days of warning before you ovulate so you can identify your fertility window and you want to confirm that ovulation did, indeed, occur. Calendar apps, basal temperature charting, and pee-on-a-stick ovulation tests don't cut it. Well-suited for PCOS women, these are the two ovulation trackers I recommend:
    - **Ovusense** (www.ovusense.com)**:** This ovulation tracker accurately monitors your core temperature. It's a medical-grade, egg-shaped device that you insert into your vagina every night. Sleep with it in there and download the information to your phone in the morning.
    - **Ovacue** (www.ovacue.com)**:** This product takes three readings every morning. A spoon-shaped oral sensor is used to take a saliva reading and a thin vaginal probe is used to take a temperature and vaginal mucus reading.

- **Scale:** You need a bathroom scale so you can weigh yourself weekly. A simple scale works just fine, but if you are going scale shopping, there are a bunch of smart scales on the market that will track your weight day-after-day for you. Be sure to get one that has a pregnancy mode because some body composition measurements may involve sending a mild electrical current through your body, and pregnant women will want to turn those features off.

- **Tape measure:** Once a week, you will measure your waist and hip circumference because those measurements are another tool for checking metabolic health. You want to get a soft, flexible tape measure designed for sewing, not a rigid one used for construction projects.

Go supplement shopping

No matter how healthy our choices are, it is impossible to live as naturally as our ancestors did. Supplements fill in the gaps and imperfections in our lifestyle and diet. They provide essential nutrients and extra support to fragile systems such as our immune system, digestive system, and reproductive system. And they can directly reduce insulin resistance and inflammation, two of the key underlying contributors to PCOS infertility.

I know this may seem like *a lot* of supplements. Think of this as a three-month supplement bootcamp that will dramatically lower systemic inflammation and improve insulin resistance. I recommend that you take all of these supplements at the recommended dosages for three months, starting Week 1 of the Fertility Fast Track (see page 68 for schedule and dosages). After that, depending on how you're doing, we may lower your dosages on some of them.

- **Berberine (BER-ber-een):** You need a 500 mg dosage. I recommend Douglas Laboratories Berberine Balance or Thorne Berberine-500. Another combination product I use is Metabolic Xtra by Pure Encapsulations. Berberine is useful for infertility because it controls blood sugar and normalizes metabolism. It facilitates weight loss, in particular visceral fat loss, and it helps lower triglyceride and cholesterol levels. Consequently, it improves pregnancy rates for PCOS women.[5,6,7]
  NOTE: If at any point you become pregnant, stop taking berberine.[8]

- **Curcumin (ker-KYOO-men):** You should take 1500 mg daily. I usually give my patients Pure Encapsulations CurcumaSorb (6 capsules daily) or Thorne Meriva 500-SF Curcumin Phytosome (3 capsules daily). This polyphenol is the active component in turmeric and is a powerful anti-inflammatory. It reduces insulin resistance and the risk of diabetes, and it lowers hypertension and protects against heart attacks. By improving your whole-body health, curcumin increases fertility and prepares your body for pregnancy.[9]
  NOTE: If at any point you become pregnant, stop taking curcumin.

- **Melatonin (mell-ah-TONE-in):** I recommend about 3 mg of melatonin per night. I like Douglas Laboratories Controlled-Release Melatonin 2 mg combined with Douglas Laboratories Melatonin 1 mg. If you have a hard time falling asleep, you may prefer the Pure Encapsulations 3 mg dose, combined with the Pure Encapsulations 0.5 mg dose. With either combo, you will take the smaller dose about two hours before you go to sleep and the larger dose at bedtime, starting in Week 3 of this program (page 96). Melatonin, a hormone that has receptors on the ovaries, increases pregnancy success rates in PCOS women.[10]

- **Myo-inositol (my-oh-in-AW-si-tall):** You should buy a bag or tub of myo-inositol powder. I recommend Pure Encapsulations Inositol (powder). You will take two scoops daily (4 grams), mixed in water. Other brands often list dosage in milligrams, not grams. 4 g equals 4000 mg. Myo-inositol is a sugar alcohol that plays a critical role in glucose metabolism. Specifically, it reduces insulin resistance, which is a central characteristic of PCOS and one of the root causes of nearly every symptom you are experiencing. Myo-inositol is more effective than metformin, a pharmaceutical insulin sensitizer, with none of metformin's side effects. Myo-inositol is so effective that among PCOS women who take this supplement daily, 70% begin having regular menstrual cycles. It improves egg quality and reduces the risk of developing gestational diabetes in pregnancy. It also reduces your lifelong risk of developing diabetes and cardiovascular disease.[11,12,13]

- **N-acetyl cysteine (en-ah-SEE-tall-siss-teen) (NAC):** I recommend 1800 mg daily of NAC and I usually give my patients Pure Encapsulations NAC 900 mg (2 capsules daily). NAC is an antioxidant. In women with PCOS, NAC improves egg quality, normalizes ovulation, and increases the chances of both getting pregnant and having a live birth. NAC supports healthy glucose metabolism and is the precursor to the production of glutathione (gloo-tuh-THEYE-own), known as the master antioxidant and detoxifier of the body. For women taking Clomid or undergoing assisted reproductive techniques, NAC improves egg quality, ovulation, pregnancy, and live birth rates. And for women with a history of preterm labor (note that all PCOS women are at increased risk of preterm labor), NAC helps you stay pregnant longer.[14,15,16,17]

- **Omega-3 fatty acids:** I recommend Pure Encapsulations O.N.E. Omega (1 softgel daily), OrthoMolecular Orthomega (2 softgels daily), or Metagenics EPA-DHA 720 (2 softgels daily). Primarily found in fatty fish, omega-3s reduce inflammation and improve immune system functioning. Our bodies need two main types, Eicosapentaenoic Acid (EPA) and Docosahexaenoic Acid (DHA). Higher blood levels of omega-3s correspond to improved female fertility and higher rates of live birth. DHA is particularly important for fetal brain development. Pregnant women who take omega-3 supplements have lower rates of preterm birth.[18,19]

- **Prenatal multivitamin:** I suggest that my patients take the Thorne Basic Prenatal (3 capsules per day) or Pure Encapsulations PreNatal Nutrients (2 capsules daily). Your prenatal multivitamin should have, at a minimum, the recommended dietary allowance (RDA) for the included vitamins and minerals. And it should have 800 to 1000 mcg (1 mg) of folate and at least 150 mcg of iodine. You should take a pharmaceutical grade multivitamin to be sure that the vitamins and minerals in the supplement are bioavailable, in a form that your body can absorb. The B vitamins should be methylated (METH-ill-ate-ed). For example, instead of folic acid, also known as vitamin B9, your multivitamin should include a folate such as methylfolate. For vitamin B12, it should have methylcobalamin, not cyanocobalamin.

- **Probiotics (pro-by-AW-ticks):** There are dozens of probiotics on the market. I like Pure Encapsulations Probiotic-5 (1 capsule daily) or Ortho Molecular Products Ortho-Biotic (1 capsule daily). Probiotics are live bacteria that benefit your gut microbiome. In women with PCOS, daily probiotics improve weight loss, triglycerides, cholesterol, and insulin resistance. They reduce testosterone levels and improve hirsutism. They also enhance mood, and in pregnancy, they reduce the risk of preeclampsia and preterm birth.[20,21,22,23]

- **Quercetin (KWAIR-si-tin):** I recommend 1000 mg daily and usually give my patients Pure Encapsulations Quercetin (4 capsules daily). Quercetin is a flavonoid found in a variety of plants, including green apples and red wine. Quercetin decreases testosterone and improves ovarian health and function. Like myo-inositol, quercetin improves insulin resistance, and additionally, it improves adiponectin (ad-i-pah-NEK-tin) receptors. Adiponectin is a hormone critical for burning fat and maintaining metabolic health. Increasing adiponectin sensitivity facilitates weight loss and maintenance.[24,25,26]

- **Vaginal probiotic:** A healthy vaginal microbiome requires adequate estrogen. Consequently, both PCOS and "hormonal" birth control disrupt the vaginal microbiome. To establish a healthy vaginal microbiome, you should take a vaginal probiotic. I recommend Women's Ther-biotic probiotic by Klaire Labs. This is an oral probiotic. Studies show that oral probiotics are very effective at establishing a healthy vaginal microbiome.[27]

- **Vitamin D3:** I recommend 2000 IU daily. I usually give my patients Pure Encapsulations Vitamin D3 1000 IU or Thorne D-1000. Be sure to check how much vitamin D is in your prenatal multivitamin (Thorne Prenatal has 1000 IU and Pure Encapsulations PreNatal has 600 IU) Don't go above 2000 IU total without discussing with your doctor. The sunshine vitamin, vitamin D is essential for blood sugar regulation, ovarian function, cancer prevention, and sleep... all things that women with PCOS struggle with. As many as 85% of women with PCOS are vitamin D deficient, and treating this deficiency improves a wide array of PCOS symptoms. Critically, women with adequate vitamin D levels have higher pregnancy rates and better pregnancy outcomes than women who are vitamin D deficient.[28,29,30,31]

Do your Sunday prep work

On Sunday, the day before each new week of the program begins, get ready for the upcoming new week.

Read the next chapter

Set aside 15 to 20 minutes on Sunday morning to read next week's chapter. This will explain what you'll be doing so you can make plans, create your weekly menu, build your weekly grocery list, shop for food and other items, and just generally get ready. You want everything in place so you set yourself up for a successful Monday.

Plan your weekly menu

At the end of each week's chapter, there is a worksheet where you can plan out that week's menu.

The Fertility Fast Track program builds on itself week after week, so in the first few weeks, you won't have complete guidance for every meal of the day. Follow the guidelines that have been given, and where there aren't guidelines, eat what you normally would.

I've found that if I give patients too many dietary recommendations all at once, they get overwhelmed and have trouble keeping everything straight.

Have faith that by the end of these 12 weeks, you will know how to eat a plant-centric, high-fiber, nutrient-dense diet.

When you read over next week's info, you'll see that you start with a daily dinner salad. That's it. That's the first dietary goal—a salad with dinner every day. Over time, you will add increasing quantities of beans, fruits, vegetables, and whole grains. And only after you are eating lots of nutritious plant-based foods for every meal of every day do we start talking about limiting meat, sugar, alcohol, gluten, and processed foods.

Start slowly, with a daily dinner salad.

If you want suggestions as you plan your meals, I've included a meal inspiration guide on page 331. Use these ideas to find recipes on the internet or in your favorite cookbook.

Build your grocery list

After you complete your weekly menu planner, you should build your Sunday grocery list. I have included items that I know you'll need, but based on the meals you plan, you'll need to add to it. In the early weeks, there will be a lot of space for your own items, but as the program progresses, I'll make more and more recommendations.

Whenever possible, I suggest that you attempt to get all of your grocery shopping for the week done in one visit. Not only will this save you time, it will reduce your opportunities to make impulse purchases.

You'll be buying lots of fruits and vegetables on this program, so it takes some planning to avoid throwing out rotten food. I recommend that you buy perishable fruits and veggies to eat Monday through Wednesday and less perishable, more durable veggies to get you through the end of the week.

Keep your pantry stocked with long-lasting nuts, seeds, beans, grains, dried fruit, pickles, and olives.

If you are strategic, you can go to the store once and make seven days worth of beautiful meals.

Go grocery shopping

Sometime on Sunday, plan to go to the grocery store.

As you progress through the Fertility Fast Track program, you'll find that you naturally do more and more of your shopping around the periphery of the grocery store. That's where the fresh produce and meat are usually located. I really only go into the inner aisles to buy dry staples such as beans, grains, nuts, and dried fruit. I also pick up some jars of pickles, olives, and tomato sauce and cooking essentials such as oils and spices.

Don't worry too much about that this week, but recognize as it happens because it is a clear sign that your diet is getting healthier.

One thing you should think about this week—organic food. I highly recommend that you buy organic produce and food products. No matter how you spin it, conventional food products contain pesticides, and pesticides are poisons. Women who are exposed to pesticides take longer to get pregnant, are more likely to miscarry, and are more likely to give birth to babies with health problems.[32]

You don't need to throw away all the non-organic foods in your kitchen, but as you buy new products, invest in organic.

Buy additional items and complete additional tasks

Some weeks, like this week, you'll have additional items to buy. I try to keep these purchases to a minimum, but sometimes, having the right tools can really improve your results.

Getting ready organizer

Here are your checklists so you are fully prepared for Day 1 of Week 1. I know it's a lot to do and buy, but you'll be so glad to get all of this out of the way. Once this is done, you'll be ready to start building healthy new habits and tackling the persistent PCOS health problems that are making you crazy.

Choose Day 1

☐ Day 1 is on _____

Make these appointments

☐ Primary care or OB-GYN appointment is on _____

☐ Specialist(s) appointment is on _____

☐ Dentist appointment is on _____

☐ Male partner's primary care appointment is on _____

Buy these health accessories

- ☐ Blood pressure cuff (prefer upper arm cuff)

- ☐ Fasting Mimicking Diet—1 (or 3) ProLon kits

- ☐ Ovulation tracker (Ovusense or Ovacue)

- ☐ Scale

- ☐ Tape measure

Buy these supplements

- ☐ Berberine (Douglas Laboratories Berberine Balance, Thorne Berberine-500, or Metabolic Xtra by Pure Encapsulations)

- ☐ Curcumin (Pure Encapsulations CurcumaSorb or Thorne Meriva 500-SF)

- ☐ Melatonin (Douglas Laboratories Controlled-Release Melatonin 2 mg with Douglas Laboratories Melatonin 1 mg or Pure Encapsulations Melatonin 3 mg with Pure Encapsulations Melatonin 0.5 mg)

- ☐ Myo-inositol powder (Pure Encapsulations Inositol (powder))

- ☐ N-acetyl cysteine (NAC) (Pure Encapsulations NAC 600 mg or 900 mg)

- ☐ Omega-3s (Pure Encapsulations O.N.E. Omega, OrthoMolecular Orthomega, or Metagenics EPA-DHA 720)

- ☐ Prenatal multivitamin (Pure Encapsulations PreNatal or Thorne Basic Prenatal)

☐ Probiotics (Pure Encapsulations Probiotic-5 *or* Ortho Molecular Products Ortho-Biotic)

☐ Quercetin (Pure Encapsulations Quercetin)

☐ Vaginal probiotic (Klaire Labs Women's Ther-biotic probiotic)

☐ Vitamin D3 (Pure Encapsulations Vitamin D3 1000 IU *or* Thorne D-1000)

Sunday planner

☐ Take your weekly measurements. (See page 325 in the workbook.)

☐ Read over Week 1's information.

☐ If you have a male partner, ask him to read the male fertility guide on page 293.

☐ Plan Week 1's meals on page 72. (See page 331 for ideas.)

☐ Build Week 1's grocery list on page 73.

☐ Go grocery shopping.

PART TWO

The 12-week Fertility Fast Track program

CHAPTER 4

Month 1, Week 1: Here we go!

*W*elcome to Week 1! This is your jump-in-and-get-started week. You are going to begin building habits that will powerfully change your health for the better. I hope that many of the habits you start this week will last for the rest of your life.

Your goals for this week are to:

1. Get into the swing of a new, healthier food schedule.
2. Eat salad.
3. Start taking your supplements.
4. Start monitoring ovulation.

You should expect that it will take a few days to figure out how to make your new schedule work for you. Don't sweat it if you're not perfect on Day 1. I'll give you some tips that have helped my patients. Try some out and see what works for you.

And stick with it. The best motivation comes from seeing results, which will honestly take a few weeks.

Only eat during the day

The first scheduling change you should implement is something called time-restricted eating. This is how you set the circadian rhythm of your digestive tract.

The basics are pretty simple. Eat breakfast, lunch, dinner, and *stop!* Divide your 24-hour day into an eating window and a fasting window. During the eating window, you can eat as much food as you'd like, but during the fasting window, don't eat anything. No dessert. No after dinner alcohol. No snacks while watching TV. Nothing that your body will recognize as food. In the evening, you can have hot tea or decaf coffee (no milk, no sugar), but that's about it.

The goal is to give your whole digestive system an overnight break, which works wonders on your metabolism and insulin resistance.

Ideally, for these first few weeks, your overnight fast should be 12 hours long. Later, you'll increase your overnight fast to 13 hours.

For most people, this means that breakfast is eaten at 7AM, shortly after waking up, and dinner is completely finished by 7PM. If your schedule is shifted by an hour or so, that's fine. The key is to finish dinner early enough that your body experiences a full 12-hour overnight fast every night.

Time-restricted eating improves metabolic markers across the board. People who limit eating to 12 or fewer day-time hours have improved insulin sensitivity, glucose tolerance, triglyceride levels, and lower blood pressure. For PCOS women, improved metabolic markers correspond with improved fertility. And pregnant women who fast for 12 hours overnight have lower fasting glucose levels, which corresponds to lower risks of gestational diabetes.[1,2,3]

Time-restricted eating is a habit that will serve you well for the rest of your life. It may take some experimentation and creative problem-solving, but find a way to have 12 food-free hours every night.

Tips:

- Schedule your eating window. Don't be vague and hand-wavy about it.
  Breakfast starts at _____
  Dinner starts at _____
  Dinner ends at _____

- If you are struggling to eat dinner early enough, try doing all of the meal prep the night before. I'll often throw a few yams in the oven for an hour and a half in the evening. While they cook, I slice and marinate raw chicken and chop salad veggies. The next day, I throw the chicken in a pan, microwave the yams, and arrange a salad for dinner in 10 minutes!

- As your body learns its new schedule, you may get hungry after dinner. Eventually, time-restricted eating reduces hunger. In the meantime, have a cup of tea or decaf coffee (no milk, no sugar). Start a fun activity that's not food related, such as an art project or a game. Or just go to bed. If you need to grab a few nuts or seeds to stop your stomach from growling, that's okay, too. And tomorrow, eat a little more at dinner![4]

- Attending evening social events is tough because they never end by 7PM. Once in a while, a late meal with friends won't harm you, but don't do this often. When social events push into your fasting window, try to finish eating as early in the evening as possible and switch to sparkling water, plain tea, or black decaf coffee. Consider extending your fast into the following morning to reach 12 hours.

- I actually don't love extending an overnight fast by pushing out breakfast too far because in the morning your cortisol levels are high (that's how you wake up). Eating lowers your cortisol, so if you skip breakfast, your cortisol stays high. And high cortisol encourages inflammation and fat storage. However, if you simply can't eat an early dinner, you can go this route and push out breakfast. Doing it this way is still better than not fasting at all.

- When you need to extend your fast on the breakfast end, you want to trick your body into thinking it's fasting when it really isn't. Do this by eating a small, high-fat, zero-sugar snack in the morning not too long after waking up. Your body will stay in fasting mode, but you'll drive down your cortisol. A handful of macadamia nuts works best as they are the highest-fat nut, but other nuts and seeds work, too. Olives are another good option. When you are on-the-go, consider the Fast Bar from ProLon (l-nutra.com/pages/fast-bar), a bar that keeps you in a fasted state while still providing your body with nourishment.

Eat a salad with dinner

From here on out, you should start dinner with a salad. Eat normally for breakfast, lunch, and dinner—we'll optimize those meals in future weeks—but before you serve your dinner entree, sit down with only salad and dressing on the table. Eat that first.

For the purpose of this book, a salad is defined as at least one and a half cups of leafy greens plus three to five different plant-based accessories. That's your base. If you want to add chicken, feta cheese, or a hardboiled egg on top of the veggies, go for it.

I recommend a salad per day for two reasons:

1. **Consistent two cups of veggies:** Humans need a lot of nutrients and fiber to be healthy. Eating vegetables (and other plants) supports every organ system and function in your body. Plus it provides essential fiber to your gut microbiome. In this Fertility Fast Track program, you will work your way up to eating six or

more cups of plants every day. A pre-dinner salad gets you one third of the way there.

2. **Nitric oxide:** Leafy greens, such as dark green lettuce, spinach, arugula, and cabbage, and other vegetables, such as beetroot, are rich in nitrates. When you eat them, your body converts them to nitric oxide, a potent antioxidant that is absolutely essential to proper immune function, cardiovascular health, and female fertility. Nitric oxide improves cervical mucus, which helps conduct sperm to egg, and then aids in implantation. In pregnancy, nitric oxide reduces the risk of preeclampsia. You get all of this by adding a salad-a-day to your diet.[5,6]

Making a salad is pretty simple. In fact, it's pretty hard to do it wrong. Basically start with a bed of greens and add what I call accessories—plant-based foods that give your salad color, flavor, texture, and nutrition. I always aim for five salad accessories, so my salads are interesting and really pack a nutritional punch. Here are some salad ingredients you should try:

- **Greens:** Buy salad greens with a rich, dark green color (not iceberg lettuce). I recommend that you buy one of those big one-pound tubs of pre-washed mixed greens every week and plan to eat it yourself. Get a second one for your partner. Each tub has about ten cups of greens in it so that makes seven salads, each with about a cup and a half of greens.

- **Fresh veggies:** Virtually any veggie that your grocery store sells will taste great on a salad. Early in the week, eat up your more perishable vegetables, such as bell peppers, cucumbers, green onions, and avocados. Then move on to longer-lasting veggies, such as cabbage, radishes, beets, celery, and carrots.

- **Fresh fruit:** Mix things up by adding chopped apple, pear, strawberry, or pomegranate.

- **Frozen veggies:** You can quickly defrost peas, corn, and soybeans by putting them in a colander and running them under cool water for a minute.

- **Veggies in a jar:** Keep olives, capers, pickled garlic, and marinated roasted bell peppers in your pantry. Choose items in glass jars, not cans (see page 115).

- **Beans and grains:** When you add beans or grains to a salad, you add fiber and protein. Your salad is more nutritious and more filling. Some of my favorite beans are lima beans, cannellini beans, and pinto beans, but really, I love them all. And for grains, I love the texture and flavor of quinoa, buckwheat, amaranth, and millet.

- **Nuts and seeds:** These are excellent salad toppers. They are full of healthy fats, vitamins, and fiber. Flax seeds are particularly healthy because they are high in vegetarian omega-3s, and some studies show that regularly eating flaxseeds improves ovulation rates and menstrual regularity. Store them in your freezer or they can go rancid.[7,8]

- **Dried fruit:** Sweeten your salad with chopped, preferably unsweetened, dried fruit. Raisins, plums, apricots, and dates are my favorites.

- **Dressing:** In terms of salad dressing, at this point, buy something natural (preferably organic) with ingredients that you recognize in a flavor you like. Use an amount that tastes good but don't drown your veggies. Consider that salad dressings can be full of sugar and fat. Personally, I love mixing high-quality olive oil and a flavorful vinegar. It's simple and delicious.

No matter what, a salad shouldn't be boring. Most days of the week, I simply put seasonal veggies on greens and enjoy. But sometimes, I like to mix things up and have a salad that feels a bit more planned. Here are some of my favorite themed salads. Start with a bed of greens.

- **Beet salad:** red beets, golden beets, green onions, strawberries, and walnuts
- **Garden salad:** tomatoes, cucumbers, bell peppers, carrots, and sunflower seeds
- **Greek salad:** cherry tomatoes, Greek olives, cucumber, artichoke hearts, and red onion
- **Taco salad:** black beans, tomatoes, avocado, corn, and white onion

Search online for salad recipes and you'll discover that you could easily eat a different salad every day of the month. Oh, and if a dinner salad isn't really your style, feel free to eat a breakfast or lunch salad instead. For more salad ideas, check out the salad inspiration list on page 333.

Eating salad is one of the best investments you can make in your health.

Tips:

- Do some of your salad prep the night before. Not all veggies hold up well to pre-chopping and fridge storage, but I've successfully stored chopped cabbage, cucumbers, carrots, bell peppers, and beets for one or more days. Chopped tomatoes, on the other hand, get slimy pretty quickly.
- To reduce veggie chopping, accessorize your salad with chop-free plants. Rinse frozen peas, corn, or soybeans in cool water to quickly defrost them. Add cherry tomatoes. Buy bags of pre-chopped veggies. Add beans or olives. Top your salad with a small handful of nuts, seeds, or dried fruit.
- Buy salad toppings from your grocery store salad bar and put them on top of your own lettuce at home.
  Buy a salad-in-a-bag kit. Obviously, fresher is better. But if a salad-in-a-bag gets a salad on your table, go for it. No one is judging your salad creativity.

Take your supplements

Get into a supplement routine. It may take a few tries to work out the kinks, but once you see how these supplements help with your PCOS symptoms, you won't be willing to go without them.

The only supplement I've recommended that absolutely needs to be taken at a specific time each day is berberine. Because it is only potent for a few hours, berberine must be taken several times throughout the day to maintain stable blood levels. It's an insulin sensitizer so it's most effective when paired with meals. Take one dose before breakfast, one dose before lunch, and one dose before dinner.

In an ideal world, you would take all of your additional supplements at their perfectly ideal times: vitamin D3 at breakfast; NAC and myo-inositol twice per day; quercetin three times per day, but never with food; and the rest at bedtime. This schedule would be a lot of work! There isn't much research showing that the significantly increased complexity caused by spacing supplements throughout the day leads to significantly better outcomes. However, complexity does make a plan like this much harder to follow.

These supplements will help you, and I want to make it as easy as possible for you to take them.

Consequently, for simplicity's sake, I recommend that during this Fertility Fast Track you take all of the supplements, except for berberine, in a big supplement binge before bedtime. The benefits of the bedtime supplement feast are:

- Most of my patients tell me that their bedtime routine is more consistent and less distracted than their morning routine. It's easier to add an extra step at night than in the morning.

- Taken with water, not juice, your supplements won't break your fast because they don't have any sugar.

- If any of them cause minor nausea, you'll sleep through it. None of these supplements should cause nausea, but everyone is different.

However, if another time of day works better for you, that's fine.

Daily supplements protocol

Here's your daily supplements protocol. You may want to dogear this page so it's easy to find.

Before Breakfast
        Berberine: 500 mg

Before Lunch
        Berberine: 500 mg

Before Dinner
        Berberine: 500 mg

Before Bed
        Mix 2 scoops of myo-inositol (4 g / 4000 mg) into a glass of water and take...
        Curcumin: 1500 mg
        NAC: 1800 mg
        Omega-3: 1 dose, which should include 600 mg EPA and 400 mg DHA
        Prenatal: 1 dose
        Probiotic: 1 dose
        Quercetin: 1000 mg
        Vaginal probiotic: 1 dose
        Vitamin D3: 2000 mg (adjust down if your prenatal already includes vitamin D)

Tips:

- It can be tough to remember to take berberine at meal time. Schedule a reminder into your phone so you don't need to remember. You can also keep your berberine with the food for each meal or at your eating location. So, keep the bottle on your kitchen table. Put one next to your coffee mug. Pack one in your lunch. If you miss a dose and remember within two hours, take it then. Otherwise, skip it and just take the next dose before the next meal as usual.

- If sorting through all of these supplements at night feels like too much work, presort them into a weekly pill sorter. Then you only have to do it once per week.

- Omega-3 supplements can cause something called fish burp, which is as unpleasant as it sounds. You'll know if you get it. If this is a problem for you, I've got two tips. First, keep your omega-3s in the freezer, and second, take them *right* before bed.

- If you want a more aggressive supplement schedule, see page 240 in Week 11. I don't recommend *everything* in the first week because I don't want to overwhelm anyone. But if you are in poor health, if you have already been trying to conceive for over a year, or if you are older than 35, it would be reasonable to start with the complete supplement schedule.

Monitor ovulation

This week, get into the habit of using your ovulation monitor, even if you currently are not ovulating. At the end of this 12-week program, you will have a detailed picture of what your ovaries are or are not doing, and that will help you make decisions regarding how to try to conceive.

Whether you chose the Ovusense or Ovacue monitor, get everything set up. Read the instructions. Install the app. And get started. Both companies have great customer service, so if you have questions or problems, contact them.

Week 1 organizer

Here are your organizer worksheets for Week 1. It may take a few days to get into the swing of things, but hopefully, by the end of this week you will have your new routines down pat and be ready for more. On Sunday, be sure to read over next week's goals and go shopping.

To-do list

☐   Buy weekly pill sorter.

Meal planner

* Fill this out on Sunday, before the start of Week 1.

	Breakfast	**Lunch**	**Dinner**	**Misc**
Mon				
Tues				
Wed				
Thurs				
Fri				
Sat				
Sun				

Grocery list

* Fill this out and go shopping on Sunday, before the start of Week 1.

☐ Greens, 1 pound carton of prewashed mixed salad greens

☐ Perishable salad veggies (avocado, bell pepper, cucumber, green onions)

☐ Durable salad veggies (tomato, carrots, celery, beets, cabbage, radishes)

☐ Frozen salad veggies (corn, peas, soybeans)

☐ Jarred veggies (olives, capers, pickled garlic, marinated roasted bell peppers)

☐ Salad fruit (apples, pears, strawberries, pomegranates)

☐ Salad nuts and seeds (flax seeds)

☐ Organic salad dressing in your favorite flavor

_____

_____

_____

_____

_____

_____

_____

_____

_____

_____

Daily checklist

* Fill in the breakfast and dinner times that support your 12-hour eating and fasting windows.

	M	T	W	Th	F	Sa	Su
Pre-breakfast berberine							
Breakfast at ____ AM							
Pre-lunch berberine							
Pre-dinner berberine							
Dinner at ____ PM							
Dinner salad							
Dinner finishes at ____ PM							
Supplements							
Ovulation monitoring							
Sunday prep for next week							

Sunday planner

☐ Take your weekly measurements. See page 325 in the workbook.

☐ Read over Week 2's information.

☐ Plan Week 2's meals on page 86. (See page 331 for ideas.)

☐ Build Week 2's grocery list on page 87.

☐ Go grocery shopping.

CHAPTER 5

Month 1, Week 2

One week ago, you started this journey. How is it going? If it's all great, great! If you are still figuring things out, that's okay, too. Every change you make gets you healthier. The closer you follow the protocol the better, but most people aren't perfect. I'm not perfect. But I always strive for better.

Whether last week was perfect or not, keep with this program. You can continue solidifying last week's routines while you add new habits.

Your goals for this week are to:

1. Make the light-dark rhythm of your life match the day-night rhythm of the earth.
2. Eat beans every day.

I know these two strategies don't exactly go together, but they are so important that I want to make sure they are at the beginning of the program. Combined, they will improve your circadian rhythm, health, mood, and gut microbiome. Make them your new normal and you'll be rewarded with improved short-term and long-term health.

And fertility. It may be hard to believe, but a strong light-dark daily rhythm and a diet that includes beans dramatically improve female fertility.

Get morning light

Your daily light-dark rhythm begins every morning when you first wake up, see the sun, and initiate something called "entrainment." This is the daily setting of your circadian rhythm. If you lived in a sunless cave, your natural circadian rhythm would be somewhere between 23.5 hours and 24.5 hours long. It probably would not be exactly 24 hours. Consequently, every single day, your circadian clock needs to be entrained, or set, to the earth's 24-hour day. Otherwise, it slowly drifts out of sync.

The light from morning sunshine goes into your eyes and triggers your optic nerves to send time-setting signals to the master clock in your brain. For entrainment to occur, your brain needs 20 to 30 minutes of sunshine when you wake up.

If the weather permits, go outside because even on a cloudy day, it's usually brighter outside than inside. And for this little bit of time, do *not* wear sunglasses. Your master clock needs to *see* the light for it to work, so you need that sunshine to go into your eyes. Don't look at the sun. That's dangerous. But for 20 to 30 minutes every morning, be in sunshine.

Additionally, if it's warm, get some sun on your skin to increase your body's production of vitamin D, nitric oxide, and other antioxidants.

Morning sunshine creates a strong circadian rhythm synchronization that causes hormonal levels across the board to start doing what they are supposed to do *when* they are supposed to do it:

- When you wake-up, levels of melatonin (sleepy hormone) go down and cortisol (wakeful hormone) go up. This makes it easier to wake up and start your day.[1]

- Morning light increases insulin sensitivity, so you can more efficiently metabolize your breakfast. Consequently, people who get bright morning light lose weight.[2,3]

- In the evening, melatonin begins to rise again. Because bright morning light shifts your circadian rhythm forward by an hour or more, people who get morning sunshine report fewer sleep disturbances. They fall asleep faster and sleep better.[4,5]

A daily morning dose of sunshine is so powerful that it boosts female fertility by one third. Women around the world are more fertile in the summer than in the winter. In a recent Dutch study, women were more likely to get pregnant if they got sunshine in the month *before* they tried to conceive. So start getting sunshine now.[6]

Morning sun exposure is one of the healthiest daily habits you can adopt. Make it a priority to set your circadian rhythm every single day. For the price of 20 to 30 minutes of morning sun, you will feel better all day long, you will enjoy better health across the board, and you will give your fertility a much needed boost.

Tips:

- Try to combine morning sunshine time with something you already do. Eat breakfast outside. Drink your coffee on the porch. Walk your dog, or just take a walk. Do a little morning gardening.

- If you can't go outside, sit in a bright, sunny window.

- If you don't live somewhere that's usually sunny in the morning, invest in a light therapy lamp, also called a light box. The standard dosage is 10,000 lux for 30 minutes. Buy a lamp that emits 10,000 lux (some are weaker) and position it about two feet from where you sit. You want the light to be slightly above your head and off to the side a bit, aimed down towards your eyes. While you eat breakfast or catch up on email, sit by your lamp for 30 minutes every morning. Make sure you use it every day because consistency is important.

- If you wear contacts or prescription glasses, check to see if the lenses provide UV protection. Scientists recently discovered that humans have UV photoreceptors in our eyes that play a role in circadian rhythm. If you get your morning sun while wearing contacts or glasses that filter out UV rays, you won't get the full benefit.[7]

- If you miss getting morning sunshine for whatever reason, get outside in the afternoon. That's great for your health and fertility as well.

Make your bedroom really dark at night

Just as your body needs morning light, it needs evening darkness. In particular, you need to sleep in a very dark room. Unless you've spent time really darkening your bedroom, it's probably not dark enough. Even a little bit of light coming through your eyelids while you sleep suppresses melatonin, raises cortisol, and disrupts your sleep quality. And that impacts your metabolism and fertility.

Nighttime melatonin is essential for the health of your ovaries and the quality of your eggs. Women's ovaries are so sensitive to the light-dark melatonin cycle that chronic exposure to light at night can actually cause infertility all on its own. And the older you are, the more sensitive you are to off-rhythm-light-induced infertility.[8]

So this week, figure out how to make your bedroom as dark as possible.[9,10]

Tips:

- Install blackout curtains or shades. Even the cheap paper blackout shades work great. The trick is to have them extend far enough past the window frame that they stop light from bleeding in around the edges.

- One night, go around your bedroom with black electrical tape and cover anything that emits light. Look for lights on chargers, powerstrips, and other electronics.

- If you have an illuminated alarm clock and you need to have an alarm clock, replace it with a touch activated clock with a red light display. (Red light doesn't suppress melatonin the way that regular white light does). Or just put a shoebox over your alarm clock and call it good. If you are in the market for a new alarm clock, read the section on dawn simulators on page 235.

- Consider using a sleep mask. This is the route I chose because it was going to be a ton of work to get my room dark enough. And on top of that, I travel frequently. It's much easier to wear a sleep mask than to run around a hotel room covering up alarm clocks, tiny lights, and whatnot.

Someway somehow, by the end of this week, make sure you are sleeping in complete darkness. The extra melatonin you produce will help you sleep better and recover from the previous day. It will nurture your ovaries and the precious eggs housed within them.

Install red night lights

In addition to your bedroom, you need to make the rest of your house nighttime friendly.

Do you have night lights in your bathroom and hallways? It's important that you can get to and from the bathroom at night without turning on any lights. Remember that light suppresses melatonin, so under normal circumstances, you want to avoid nighttime light.

All light at night is bad. No matter what color it is, it raises your cortisol level, which wakes you up. But if you need a little light to get to the bathroom, red light is the least bad. Unlike normal light bulbs, which cause melatonin levels to plummet, red light bulbs have only a minimal effect on melatonin. So after a short nighttime trip, you'll be able to fall back to sleep much more easily and your body (including your eggs) will get the melatonin it needs.[11]

> ### Sleeping with a night light
>
> If you or your partner are one of the 15% of adults who are afraid of the dark, you might not be able to sleep comfortably in the dark. Put a red night light in your bedroom to avoid suppressing melatonin, and try sleeping with a sleep mask to encourage a healthy nighttime cortisol dip.[12]

Eat some beans every single day

Beans are one of the most nutritious foods you can add to your diet. They are full of nutrients and fiber that nurture your body and your gut microbiome.

Beans and lentils lower post-meal glucose levels, which means that they decrease post-meal blood sugar spikes and improve insulin functioning. Additionally, they keep your blood sugar stable all the way up to your next meal, enabling you to reduce snacking without that low-blood-sugar feeling.[13]

And they improve fertility! Beans are rich in a variety of nutrients, including iron and manganese, that are essential for normal ovulation. Women who eat more vegetable protein, such as beans and legumes, and less meat have an easier time getting pregnant.[14]

Starting this week, eat half a cup of beans or lentils at some point every day. In a couple of weeks, you will increase this to a full cup, but if you start at half a cup, your digestive tract can adjust to the increase in fiber slowly.

Tips:

- When in doubt, toss half a cup of beans on your dinner salad. Chickpeas, cannellini beans, and lima beans are excellent salad beans. This is by far the easiest way to add half a cup of beans to your day.

- Bean spreads are great in sandwiches. There's hummus, which is made from chickpeas and tahini. But you can make a delicious spread from pretty much any type of bean. Do an internet search for some tasty recipes.

- Peanuts are legumes, and organic, chunky, sugar-free peanut butter is an excellent source of fiber. While I don't think it would be pleasant to try and eat half cup of peanut butter, a tablespoon or two is a healthy way to add more beans to your diet. Eat it with apples or bananas, or fix yourself an old-fashioned "ants on a log" (celery stick smeared with peanut butter, topped with raisins in a row).

- Consider experimenting with beans at breakfast. An added benefit of having beans with your coffee is that your blood glucose will be stable through lunch so you'll feel better all morning. Plus, next week, you are going to start eating more of your calories earlier in the day. Beans at breakfast are a great way to make breakfast a heartier, more satisfying meal. Some bean-friendly breakfasts to explore:

- **Black bean scramble:** black beans, mushrooms, and onions scrambled with eggs
- **Breakfast tacos:** beans, scrambled eggs, avocado, and salsa in corn tortillas
- **Cowboy breakfast:** beans, potatoes, and corn, cooked in a cast iron skillet
- **English breakfast:** British baked beans (which are much less sweet than American baked beans), turkey sausage, and grilled tomatoes
- **Huevos rancheros:** refried beans topped with a fried egg, avocado, and salsa
- **Hummus and avocado bowl**

For more recipe ideas, check out the menu inspirations on page 331.

Week 2 organizer

And that's it for Week 2. Sunlight in the morning. Darkness at night. And half a cup of beans sometime every day. Here are your checklists to get you going.

To-do list

* You may not need to do everything on this list to get all of the evening darkness you require. Make the changes you need for your specific situation.

☐ Buy 10,000 lux light therapy lamp.

☐ Hang blackout curtains or shades.

☐ Replace alarm clock with touch-activated alarm clock (or a dawn simulator, page 235).

☐ Use black electrical tape to cover any tiny lights in your bedroom.

☐ Sleep with a sleep mask.

☐ Install red night lights.

Meal planner

* Fill this out on Sunday of Week 1, before the start of Week 2. Remember to include ½ cup of beans per day.

	Breakfast	Lunch	Dinner	Misc
Mon				
Tues				
Wed				
Thurs				
Fri				
Sat				
Sun				

Grocery list

* Fill this out and go shopping on Sunday of Week 1, before the start of Week 2.

- ☐ Greens, 1 pound carton of prewashed mixed salad greens

- ☐ Perishable salad veggies (avocado, bell pepper, cucumber, green onions)

- ☐ Durable salad veggies (tomato, carrots, celery, beets, cabbage, radishes)

- ☐ Frozen salad veggies (corn, peas, soybeans)

- ☐ Jarred veggies (olives, capers, pickled garlic, marinated roasted bell peppers)

- ☐ Salad fruit (apples, pears, strawberries, pomegranate)

- ☐ Salad nuts and seeds

- ☐ Organic salad dressing in your favorite flavor

- ☐ 3 cans of beans or 1 pound of dried beans, any type

_____

_____

_____

_____

_____

_____

_____

_____

Daily checklist

	M	T	W	Th	F	Sa	Su
Eat ½ cup of beans, anytime							
Pre-breakfast berberine							
Breakfast at _____ AM							
Morning sunshine, 20-30 minutes							
Pre-lunch berberine							
Pre-dinner berberine							
Dinner at _____ PM							
Dinner salad							
Dinner finishes at _____ PM							
Supplements							
Ovulation monitoring							
Sunday prep for next week							

Sunday planner

☐ Take your weekly measurements. See page 325 in the workbook.

☐ Read over Week 3's information.

☐ Plan Week 3's meals on page 102. (See page 331 for ideas.)

☐ Build Week 3's grocery list on page 103.

☐ Go grocery shopping.

☐ Double check that you have melatonin because you'll start using it next week. (Douglas Laboratories Controlled-Release Melatonin 2 mg *with* Douglas Laboratories Melatonin 1 mg *or* Pure Encapsulations Melatonin 3 mg *with* Pure Encapsulations Melatonin 0.5 mg)

☐ Make sure your first ProLon box has arrived because you've got just one week before your first Fasting Mimicking Diet.

☐ Make sure you have your doctor's approval to do the Fasting Mimicking Diet, and if you have any health conditions, make sure you are fasting under the supervision of a healthcare provider.

CHAPTER 6

Month 1, Week 3

 *T*his week, you'll continue to shift your schedule to align with a natural circadian rhythm. The two main goals are to:

1. At night, sleep at the right time and for the right amount of time.
2. During the day, eat a big breakfast, a moderate lunch, and a small dinner.

Although it may not be instantly obvious, these two strategies support each other because they are the last two big pieces of the circadian puzzle. When you get proper sleep, you feel pretty hungry shortly after waking up. You naturally eat a big breakfast to fuel the activities of the upcoming day. And by the time evening rolls around, you are ready for a light dinner, some quiet activity, and bed.

That's the rhythm that our ancestors lived by. That's the rhythm you need to recreate.

Set a sleeping window

In the same way that you now have eating and fasting windows, you also need a sleeping window.

Sleep is one-third of our circadian rhythm and its primary purpose is rejuvenation. Good sleep facilitates thinking and learning, restores your body's resiliency, and is foundational to good health. Not surprisingly, good sleep promotes fertility, and disrupted or short sleep is an independent risk factor for infertility.

Scientists often study the effects of poor sleep and disrupted circadian rhythm by focusing on shift workers, women who work at night and, as a result, sleep during the day. Even if they only work part of the night or work late only a few days a week, these shift workers experience much higher rates of infertility, miscarriage, and preterm delivery than their daytime working counterparts. There are three contributing factors to the shift work–infertility link, and they all apply to PCOS as well.[1]

1. Shift workers often sleep less than the recommended seven to eight hours, and women who sleep less are more likely to experience menstrual irregularity and infertility.[2]

2. Off-schedule sleep, even if it only happens once or twice per week, disrupts circadian rhythm and increases insulin resistance and metabolic disorder, which causes menstrual irregularity.[3]

3. Disrupted circadian rhythm leads to poorer sleep quality, and any form of sleep disturbance lowers melatonin levels. Your eggs and ovaries have melatonin receptors. Disrupted melatonin production damages your eggs, decreases your chances of getting pregnant, and increases your chances of a miscarriage.[4]

Like shift workers, PCOS women often sleep poorly for too few hours and experience shifted circadian rhythms. Most of us have some degree of delayed sleep phase syndrome (DSPS)—our whole sleep-wake cycle runs late and we are night owls. We go to bed late, and we're not actually done sleeping when it's time to get up in the morning. We also have higher rates of sleep apnea (AP-nee-ah), a form of disordered breathing that causes frequent waking.[5,6,7]

> ### Sleep apnea
>
> Make sure you discuss sleep apnea with your primary care physician, and if you've never been screened, discuss your risk factors and whether you should get tested. Sleep apnea causes elevated levels of the hormone prolactin. High prolactin, also known as hyperprolactinemia (hy-per-pro-lak-teh-NEE-mee-ah), causes infertility. Women who treat sleep apnea with continuous positive airway pressure (CPAP) therapy experience a dramatic drop in prolactin, which improves fertility.[8]

For women with PCOS, getting good sleep is hard. It doesn't just happen. You have to plan for it. Your sleep cycle actually begins in the morning when you wake up and get a solid dose of morning sunshine. That triggers the beginning of your 24-hour melatonin and cortisol cycles. Keep prioritizing this.

The next step is to get on a strict schedule. For optimal health, you need seven to eight hours of sleep every single night. Any more or less is associated with poor health. That means you should commit to being in bed, lights out for eight hours nightly, even on weekends and holidays.

The schedule most of my patients settle on is bedtime between 10PM and 11PM and wake-up at 7AM. You can shift it earlier if you need to, but try not to shift later.

Tips:

- Just like you set your eating window, set your sleeping window:
  Wake up at _____
  Bedtime routine starts at _____
  In bed at _____

- Set an alarm on your phone or another device that alerts you when it's time to start getting ready for bed.

- If you use area lamps in the evening (which you should, see page 95), put them on timers so they turn off at bedtime.

- Get smart bulbs for overhead lighting and program them to dim in the evening and turn off at bedtime.

- On weekends, don't stay up late and sleep in. This is called social jet lag. When you shift your sleep schedule on the weekend, your body experiences this as traveling across time zones. Just like real jet lag, social jet lag wreaks havoc on your circadian rhythm. Weekend social jet lag doubles your risk of diabetes and metabolic syndrome. So try to keep the same sleep rhythm, even on the weekends.[9]

- In the mornings, set a gentle alarm that doesn't jolt you awake. Consider using a dawn simulator (page 235). Have it go off at the same time every day, even on weekends.

- If you must work at night, understand that nothing can completely undo the stress that this puts on your body. But the more you can simulate a natural light-dark cycle that corresponds to your shifted schedule, the better. Try to maintain your shifted schedule even on your days off.

Practice good sleep hygiene

Your body starts preparing for sleep several hours before you actually go to bed. Under natural lighting conditions, your body begins producing melatonin around sunset. The amount of melatonin in your bloodstream slowly increases, reaching its peak at 2AM. Then, melatonin levels slowly fall as your body transitions to morning.

Sleep hygiene is your chosen bedtime and sleep routines that support restorative sleep.

Good sleep hygiene starts around dinner time when natural light begins to fade. In general, you want to mimic outside lighting conditions inside your home. Dim indoor lighting and avoid bright screens. Give your body time to wind down and prepare for sleep.

And then, when you go to bed, go to sleep. Your bed should only be for sleeping and sex. If you want to read or watch TV (not before bed!), go do it somewhere else.

Last week, you made your bedroom dark. You should also keep it cool, between 60 and 67 degrees Fahrenheit. Get a bedside fan so you can cool off if you get hot.

Use gentle white noise to block out environmental noises. You can find a free app for your phone, or just run your fan all night if it's not too loud.

Make your bedroom a dark, cool, relaxing place to sleep.

Tips:
- Dim the lights around sunset. If you can, switch to table and floor lamps and outfit them with warm-toned bulbs. All light bulbs have a Kelvin rating indicating color temperature. Higher numbers, for example 5000 Kelvins, are daylight blue. For evening lamps, choose bulbs with lower Kelvin ratings, around 2700 or less. Sometimes called "soft white" or "warm white," these bulbs emit light on the

warmer end of the color spectrum and allow your body to begin producing melatonin.

- Start relaxing a good two hours before bed. Have a cup of herbal tea. Read a book. Work on a craft or hobby. Even some housework like folding laundry and washing dishes can be repetitive and meditative.

- Avoid screens two hours before bed. This includes televisions, computers, tablets, and smartphones. Screens are bright and usually emit significant blue light, which wakes you up and suppresses melatonin. If you need to do computer work, make sure you dim your screen and enable night shift or dark mode to filter out some of the blue light.

- Consider a relaxing hot bath before bed. Add a cup of epsom salts and 15 drops of organic lavender essential oil. This is my personal nighttime sedative and it works its wonders every time.

Take melatonin

When it comes to infertility, melatonin is a surprising powerhouse supplement that improves sleep and egg quality simultaneously.

PCOS women respond particularly well to melatonin supplements. Of course, it helps us fall asleep faster, sleep longer, and sleep better. But the benefits for PCOS women extend beyond sleep. Melatonin supplements improve the health of our ovaries and increase our estrogen levels, and this improves everything related to PCOS, including our fertility. In a recent study, PCOS women who took 2 mg of melatonin at bedtime for 6 months menstruated more regularly, had improved egg quality, and experienced a marked reduction in testosterone levels.[10,11,12,13,14]

In another study of PCOS women undergoing IVF, those who took 3 mg of melatonin combined with 4 g of myo-inositol produced much higher quality eggs and embryos than those who took myo-inositol without melatonin.[15]

To get the best sleep and fertility results, take melatonin twice per evening—a small dose about two hours before bedtime and a slightly larger dose at bedtime.

The first smaller dose enhances your body's transition into sleep mode. I recommend 0.5 to 1 mg around 8PM. This low dose mimics your natural melatonin cycle. It's the safest, least habit-forming, and most effective way to give your melatonin cycle a little nudge to get things going.[16]

It should make you really tired around 10PM (assuming you don't counteract it with bright light from light bulbs and screens). If you get too tired too early, you can push this first dose back to 9PM or even 9:30PM.

Then, at bedtime, take another slightly larger dose. For most of my patients, I recommend Douglas Laboratories Controlled-Release Melatonin 2 mg, which will help you maintain melatonin levels through the first part of the night. At around 2AM when the supplement runs out, your natural melatonin levels also begin to drop as your body transitions into the morning wake-up part of the melatonin cycle.

If you sometimes have trouble falling asleep, you might prefer the 3 mg dose of melatonin from Pure Encapsulations at bedtime. This instant release formula will amplify your sleep cues and help you drift off to sleep.

Tips:
- The 1 mg tablets from Douglas Laboratories are chewable, so you can keep a few by your bed and grab an extra for those nights when you need a little more help falling asleep. This may be the case if your new sleep schedule is earlier than your previous sleep schedule.

- I do not recommend taking high-dose melatonin. Melatonin is a hormone, and its health benefits come from having the right amount at the right time. More is not better. In fact, too much melatonin will *disrupt* your melatonin cycle and could actually stop ovulation. Unless your doctor recommends it, don't take more than 5 mg in a single night.[17]

- Traveling causes acute circadian rhythm dysfunction. I get this all of the time because I lecture around the world. This is the one situation where I recommend a very short, higher dose of melatonin. On your first evening in a new time zone, take 5 mg of melatonin at your normal bedtime in the new time zone. Make sure you take a supplement that is instant release, not timed release or sustained release. I recommend Thorne Melaton-5. Take the 5 mg bedtime dose for three nights in a row to reset your clock quickly. Repeat this process when you return home.[18]

Eat a bigger breakfast and a smaller dinner

The last habit for this week is to start working on what's called "caloric timing." In the United States, most people eat a small breakfast or skip it altogether, then a big lunch, followed by an even bigger dinner. This is totally backwards from how our bodies are designed to eat. Breakfast should be your biggest meal of the day, and dinner should be your smallest.

Your body is actually more insulin sensitive and more capable of properly metabolizing food in the morning. This means that the food you eat in the morning is more likely to get used as fuel, whereas food you eat in the evenings is more likely to get stored as fat.[19]

There was an incredible study where researchers took two groups of obese women and fed them exactly the same diet. In one group, the women ate half of their calories for breakfast, a third of their calories for lunch, and then a very light dinner. In the other group, the participants flipped this caloric schedule. They ate a very light breakfast, a third of their calories for lunch, and half of their calories for dinner. They consumed exactly the same foods, just swapped breakfast and dinner between the two groups.

Both groups lost weight, but the women who ate half of their calories for breakfast lost 2.5 times more weight just by eating their biggest meal in the morning instead of at night. And a ton of it was visceral belly fat. Additionally, the big breakfast group had better insulin levels, lower triglyceride levels (which is good), no post-meal glucose spikes (also good), and they felt less hungry all day because they had lower levels of ghrelin (a hunger hormone, also good).[20]

This same team of researchers did another nearly identical study with PCOS women. After 90 days of following a big-breakfast-small-dinner schedule, women with PCOS experienced a 56% decrease in insulin resistance, a 50% decrease in testosterone, and a 50% *increase* in ovulation.[21]

The big-breakfast-small-dinner schedule also lowers systemic inflammation, and because nighttime eating disrupts sleep, nixing late night snacks improves sleep quality.[22]

Tips:

- Your goal is not to eat less. You are just shifting more of your food away from dinner and into breakfast.

- Consider swapping your meals. Eat what you'd normally eat for dinner at breakfast time and eat your breakfast for dinner. Try chicken, roasted veggies, and a sweet potato for breakfast and a salad followed by a 2-egg veggie omelet for dinner.

- You may not be able to make this change in a day. To shift your calories earlier in the day without upsetting your stomach, take a week or two and slowly begin eating more for breakfast and less for dinner.

- Add extra fruit, veggies, and beans, plus an egg to your breakfast. For example, eat your normal breakfast, whatever that is, plus half a cup of beans topped with an egg and a piece of fruit to create a substantial meal.

- By eating a hearty breakfast, eventually you'll naturally be less hungry at dinner. Make sure you pay attention to your hunger cues. Start dinner with less food on your plate, eat slowly, and only take more food if you are hungry. This change takes time.

See page 332 for more satisfying breakfast meal options and recommendations for light, enjoyable dinners.

Week 3 organizer

That's Week 3. Focus primarily on sleep and start eating a heartier breakfast plus a smaller dinner. Both sleep and hunger are time-dependent habits that change slowly. That's the good and the bad news. Because sleep and hunger are deeply ingrained and triggered by timed hormones, they change slowly. But they do change, and once they are solidly fixed at new, healthier times, they tend to stick with minimal effort.

To-do list

- ☐ Implement evening dim light solution (area lamps with warm bulbs or smart bulbs).

- ☐ Buy a small bedside table fan, for temperature control and white noise.

- ☐ Set a bedtime alarm to remind you to get to bed on time.

- ☐ Put home lights on bedtime timers.

- ☐ Install a white noise app on your phone.

Meal planner

* Fill this out on Sunday of Week 2, before the start of Week 3. Remember that breakfast should be the biggest meal of the day and dinner should be the smallest.

	Breakfast	Lunch	Dinner	Misc
Mon				
Tues				
Wed				
Thurs				
Fri				
Sat				
Sun				

Grocery list

* Fill this out and go shopping on Sunday of Week 2, before the start of Week 3.

☐ Greens, 1 pound carton of prewashed mixed salad greens

☐ Salad accessories (veggies, fruits, nuts, dressing)

☐ 3 cans of beans or 1 pound of dried beans, any type

_____

_____

_____

_____

_____

_____

_____

_____

_____

_____

_____

_____

_____

_____

_____

_____

_____

Daily checklist

* I know this list is starting to get long. If it feels overwhelming, remember that most of these habits are quick, like downing a supplement, or they are simply putting a time on something you have to do anyway, like dinnertime and bedtime. The goal of the checklist is to help you remember all of these little pieces, not to make you crazy.

	M	T	W	Th	F	Sa	Su
Eat ½ cup of beans, anytime							
Wake up at _____ AM							
Pre-breakfast berberine							
Breakfast at _____ AM, biggest meal of the day							
Morning sunshine, 20-30 minutes							
Pre-lunch berberine							
Lunch, medium meal of the day							
Pre-dinner berberine							
Dinner at _____ PM, smallest meal of the day							
Dinner salad							
Dinner finishes at _____ PM							
Switch to evening, dim-light mode at _____ PM							
Take melatonin, 1 mg, about 2 hours before bed							
Supplements							
Take melatonin, 2 mg, right at bedtime							
In bed at _____ PM							
Ovulation monitoring							
Sunday prep for next week							

Sunday planner

☐ Take your weekly measurements. See page 325 in the workbook.

☐ Read over next week's information.

☐ Review the information in your ProLon box.

☐ Put your five fasting days on your calendar. I recommend Monday through Friday so you can celebrate your success on the weekend, but pick whichever five days work best for you, recognizing that the first two to three days will be the hardest.

☐ Plan Week 4's meals on page 124. (See page 331 for ideas.)

☐ Build Week 4's grocery list on page 125.

☐ Go grocery shopping (You can either go shopping on Sunday and buy items that will last until you finish your fast or postpone grocery shopping by a few days so your food doesn't go bad).

CHAPTER 7

Month 1, Week 4: Fasting

*T*his week is your first fasting week! I'm so excited for you. Fasting is a transformative experience. By this time next week, you will feel great!

Right now, if you're nervous, that's okay. I was nervous about my first fast, too. I worried that I'd be hungry and irritable and that I wouldn't be able to concentrate properly. While I was a little hungry during the first few days, it wasn't too bad. I maintained my normal work schedule just fine, and by Day 3, I had more energy than I normally do.

Since that initial fast, I've done 15 additional fasts, and I've guided numerous women through ProLon fasts. Because this diet mimics fasting and is not a true water fast, negative experiences are rare, and most women find that the benefits (weight loss, enhanced metabolism, and improved health markers like cholesterol, blood sugar, and blood pressure) far outweigh any of the challenges they encounter.

I love food, but much to my surprise, I've learned that I also love fasting (or at least fasting mimicking). It's liberating to have almost a whole week's worth of tiny meals planned out, and it's amazing how much extra time there is in a day when you don't prepare and sit down to three substantial meals. I look forward to my ProLon weeks because I am so much more productive.

A fasting week is a great time to tackle large projects. During each fasting week of this Fertility Fast Track program, I will show you how to remove dangerous chemicals from part of your home. I always recommend that my patients start with their kitchen because it's the biggest job and reaps the most health benefits. Your goals for the next few days are to:

1. Fast. Especially for the first few days of this week, focus on your fast.
2. Get plastics, pesticides, and other toxic chemicals out of your kitchen.

Creating a healthy living space is a long process, but it's one that is vitally important for your long-term health and the health of your family. Most of the toxins in our bodies enter through the food and beverages we consume, so the kitchen is the first room in your home that should go green.

Fast for five days

On Monday, or whatever day works best for you, start your fast. It's pretty straightforward and there isn't much preparation. Just eat the food that's provided in your ProLon kit on the schedule provided by ProLon.

While you do the fast, hit pause on your supplement routine. Take a break from the berberine and the bedtime supplement smorgasbord. The only supplement you should continue taking is melatonin to support your new sleep habit.

Tips:

- Plan for a mellow week if you can. For most people, the first two to three days are the hardest. Day 3 can be particularly challenging for women with PCOS on their first five-day fast. Typically, sometime on Day 3, your body runs out of sugar and must switch to burning fat, a process called ketosis. If your body has been in sugar-burning, fat-storage mode for a long time, your body may struggle with this switch. For a few hours, you may feel hungry and jittery. Don't cheat on the fast. Once your body makes the switch, you'll feel great. I promise. Hydrate with the teas and the power drink included, and take a walk. The hunger will pass and when it does, your body will be burning fat, possibly for the first time in a long while.

- Drink a lot. The included teas, the power drink, and water are all great.

- Avoid strenuous physical activity while fasting. Walking and easy yoga are fine so long as you feel good.

- Follow an early bedtime schedule this week. It's likely going to be what your body wants.

- On Saturday, or whenever your first post-fast day is, ease back into eating. Start with light soups, fruit, a small serving of beans, and other plant-based foods.

- Plan to celebrate your success with a fancy Sunday brunch. I like to have a nice steak or wild shrimp with yams, an elaborate fruit salad, and a small virgin mimosa (orange juice mixed with lemon sparkling water).

Buy organic from here on out

When you finish your fast and ease back into eating, you will have a new perspective on food. Truly. Take advantage of this by deeply reconsidering the quality of the foods you typically eat. Food is the fuel that maintains this extraordinary body that you live in. The food you eat becomes your skin, your bones, and your brain. If you get pregnant, the food you eat becomes your baby.

When you eat food tainted with pesticides and industrial chemicals, those toxic substances are incorporated into your body and your baby.

If you haven't already, now is the time to switch to organic food.

In particular, after your fast, it is absolutely essential to eat clean, organic food. During these days, your body will switch on stem cells and begin rapid cell rejuvenation. This is a period of increased susceptibility to endocrine disruptors, industrial chemicals, and toxins.

It's extremely hard to buy 100% of your food organic. Even the fanciest grocery stores don't usually have organic versions of everything. And sometimes, the organic version is double or triple the price of the conventional option. It's crazy!

Everyone's lifestyle and budget are different, so you'll need to find the food buying strategies that work for you. In general, buy the healthiest and most natural foods you can afford.

Tips:

- If buying all organic foods is simply not in your budget, prioritize buying organic when it comes to the "dirty dozen," the fruits and vegetables most contaminated with pesticides according to the Environmental Working Group, a non-profit environmental health organization. The 2019 list is, in order of most to least contaminated: strawberries, spinach, kale, nectarines, apples, grapes, peaches, cherries, pears, tomatoes, celery, and potatoes. You can find the up-to-date list at www.ewg.org/foodnews/dirty-dozen.php.

- I always buy organic when it comes to flours, grains, and beans because these crops can have high levels of the herbicide glyphosate (a key ingredient in Roundup). At the end of the growing season, farmers actually spray glyphosate on their crops to kill them. This practice causes grain and bean crops to dry quickly and uniformly so they can be harvested earlier. It also dramatically increases the amount of herbicide residue on these foods.

- Meat, eggs, and dairy should be organic and pasture-raised. At the very least, they should be antibiotic-free.

- Fish should be wild and sustainably harvested, or, again, at least antibiotic free. Stay away from large fish, such as swordfish, tuna, shark, tilefish, and king mackerel, because they are high in mercury and other heavy metals.

- If you think about price per nutrient, not price per calorie, packaged foods, such as crackers, breakfast cereals, and chips, are the biggest rip-off in the grocery store, especially when they are organic. You are paying for the box, plastic, and advertising campaign. And usually, all you get are flour, sugar, salt, and oil baked in a fancy shape. Buy more fruits and vegetables and fewer processed grain products. Unprocessed foods are healthier and a better deal.

- Save money and improve your health by cutting out juices, sodas, and alcohol. They are expensive and don't provide you with any nutrition. In fact, they increase gut microbiome problems, fatty liver, and insulin resistance. If you like flavored drinks, try herbal teas and water with a squirt of lemon. They are healthier and more economical options.

Get plastic out of your kitchen and away from your food

Once you start buying organic food, you need to make sure that you don't introduce synthetic chemicals during cooking and storage. One of the most important long-term changes you can make is to switch away from plastic in your kitchen.

Plastic looks solid, like glass or metal, but the molecules that make up plastic have a tendency to migrate. Think about that new vinyl smell or the taste of a bottle of water that's been left in the sun. You can smell and taste plastic because plastic releases chemicals into surrounding air and water. When plastic touches your food, it releases chemicals into your food.

Plastics contain endocrine disruptors such as bisphenol A (BPA) and phthalates. These chemicals are estrogen-mimickers. They fit into the estrogen receptors throughout your body, but because they aren't real estrogen, they trigger dysfunctional behaviors in your cells.

Women with PCOS already have low estrogen levels. Estrogen-mimickers like BPA make PCOS much worse. BPA is linked to higher testosterone levels, which exacerbates acne, hirsutism, and thinning hair. BPA causes obesity and increases your risk of diabetes and metabolic disorder.[1,2,3,4]

The female reproductive system is richly populated with estrogen receptors, so it's not surprising that infertile women generally have higher blood levels of BPA than fertile women. BPA and other endocrine disruptors cause female infertility by altering reproductive hormone levels and changing the way reproductive organs function. Specifically, BPA changes the way uterine cells behave, interfering with the ability of a fertilized egg to implant in the uterine wall.[5,6]

If a woman does get pregnant, BPA and other endocrine disruptors harm her developing baby. These chemicals cross the placenta and accumulate in the fetus, impacting the development of the baby's brain, reproductive organs, and all of her metabolic pathways. Children exposed to endocrine disruptors while in the womb are more likely to become obese. BPA alters the hypothalamus in the brain, causing permanent circadian rhythm disruption and hyperactivity. Children exposed to BPA in utero are more likely to exhibit disruptive behaviors and are at greater risk of depression. Breast tissue responds to BPA so children exposed to BPA also have a higher risk of developing breast cancer as adults.[7,8]

And on top of all that, in girl children, BPA causes PCOS. In fact, when scientists want to study PCOS in rats, they can induce PCOS by exposing rat fetuses to environmentally relevant levels of BPA.[9]

The BPA-PCOS link is so strong that women with PCOS have, on average, blood levels of BPA that are about three times higher than non-PCOS women.[10,11]

As I've mentioned, one of the best ways to limit your exposure to BPA, phthalates, and other endocrine disruptors is to keep plastic away from your food. These chemicals leach out of plastic bottles, melamine plates, nylon spatulas, and tupperware into your food.

This week, go through your kitchen and, first, find all of the plastic.

Here are some places to look:

- **Drink containers:** Do you carry around a water bottle or coffee thermos? There are no safe plastic options here. Opt for glass or stainless steel.

- **Food storage containers:** How do you store leftovers? If you use plastic tupperware, plastic bags, and plastic wrap, you should switch to glass, stainless steel, and silicone containers. You can also wrap food in aluminum foil.

- **Cooking utensils:** What materials are your spatulas, ladles, and spoons made from? Black nylon is plastic. Wood, metal, and silicone are all safer options.

- **Pots and pans:** For cookware, go with ceramic, stainless steel, enamel, or cast iron. Although not exactly plastic, the plasma perfluoroalkyl substances (PFASs) used in most nonstick cookware and other nonstick items are linked to metabolic disorders in women.[12]

- **Eatingware:** Are your cups or plates plastic? All of your dishes and drinkware should be ceramic or glass. If you want something breakproof, try enamelware.

- **Microwave plate cover:** What do you cover your food with when you microwave it? Never, never, never put any type of plastic in the microwave, even if it says it is microwave safe. (These "safe" items won't melt, but they still leach chemicals into your food.) You can buy a glass microwave plate cover. I happen to have an all-glass domed pot lid that works great. Glass pie pans and paper towels also work.

- **Small electric appliances:** Water kettles, coffee makers, blenders, food processors, yogurt makers—they are almost all plastic! Whenever you can, choose items that are glass or stainless steel.

- **Miscellaneous items:** Keep looking. What about your colander, butter dish, mixing bowls, and measuring cups? If it touches food, especially hot food, it shouldn't be plastic. Mixing bowls need to be metal because if you use a hand mixer in a plastic bowl, you'll scrape tiny pieces of plastic into whatever you are mixing.

Replacing all of this plastic in one week would be a monumental and expensive undertaking. The next thing to do is prioritize.

1. **Items that combine food, plastic, and heat.** Heat increases the rate that plasticizers migrate from plastic into food. So, the first items you should replace are cooking utensils, plates, mugs, thermoses, colanders, and microwave plate covers.

2. **Items in contact with food or beverages for extended times.** This includes your water bottle and your tupperware. Chemicals leach more quickly into fatty foods than other types of food, so if you have a plastic butter dish, that should also be high on your list.

3. **Appliances that use heat, especially ones you use frequently.** If you use a drip coffeemaker every morning, you should seriously consider replacing it with a plastic-free option. Percolators,

French presses, and pour overs are often 100% stainless steel and/or glass.

4. Plastic items that you rarely use or that you only use with cold, dry ingredients are fine to keep. Don't worry about your salad spinner, measuring spoons, popsicle molds, ice cube trays, cookie cutters, and things like that.

Tips:

- Grab a bag. When you find something plastic that you are ready to part with, throw it in the bag and add it to a "replace this" list. Donate the bag right away.

- Thrift stores and estate sales are often overflowing with older, plastic-free kitchen items. If you need to replace a lot of kitchenware, you can save significant money by buying used.

- Make sure you know how to use and clean your new non-plastic items. Wood cannot go in the dishwasher. It's safe to gently scrub most metal items with a metal scouring pad. Tempered glass can usually withstand rapid temperature changes, but it's still not a good idea to throw hot glass in the sink. It could shatter.

Stop buying food in plastic containers and cans (when possible)

As you go through your kitchen, you'll likely notice that a significant percentage of the plastic you find comes from the grocery store in the form of food packaging. Next time you go grocery shopping, in addition to choosing organic, choose items with less packaging.

In general, food packaging is bad news. Packaged foods are almost always less healthy than fresh, unpackaged foods. Packaging is terrible for the environment. And, the chemicals in food packaging, especially in plastics and cans, migrate into the food we eat.

When you can, avoid plastic. Because plastics are absorbed by fats, plastic-wrapped meats and dairy items are the worst. Peanut butter, oil, butter spreads, mayonnaise, and other high-fat items should also be in plastic-free containers. On the other hand, don't worry about fresh produce, cold items, and dry items, which are less likely to be plastic-contaminated, even when they are sold in plastic bags or clamshells. Bagged salad, clamshells of berries, bags of rice, beans, and crackers—the packaging shouldn't leach in these cases.

Cans are another type of food packaging to avoid. Virtually all cans are lined with a resin that contains BPA. Most cans that say "BPA-free" contain Bisphenol S (BPS) or Bisphenol F (BPF), sister chemicals that are just as endocrine-disrupting as BPA but less famous and less regulated.

When you buy convenience foods, you can avoid BPA, phthalates, and other endocrine disruptors by choosing some of these great options:

- **Glass:** If you ever need to choose between something in plastic, in a can, or in glass, choose glass. I buy all sorts of items in glass—tomato sauce, olives, peanut butter, mustard, cooking oil, and salad dressing, just to name a few.

- **Frozen:** Instead of canned fruits and veggies, choose frozen. Yes, they come in a plastic bag, but they go in frozen and stay frozen, so they don't leach.

- **Tetra Pak boxes:** These cardboard boxes are lined with polyethylene plastic and aluminum, and in tests, they don't seem to leach. They are a reasonable alternative to cans for soups, broths, stewed tomatoes, and beans.

- **Dried:** Beans, soups, sauces, and pastas are usually available dried. Cook them yourself from scratch for a meal that is healthier and better tasting than the canned version.

- **Some cans:** If you are willing to do *a lot* of research, a few brands have replaced their can linings with bisphenol-free liners. The Environmental Working Group's report on canned foods is a good place to start: www.ewg.org/research/bpa-canned-food. I feel comfortable eating canned foods from Eden Organic and Amy's.

- **Don't buy it:** For items that are hard to find plastic free, consider simply eating less or avoiding them altogether. These would be items like cheese, lunch meat, and yogurt.

Learning how to food shop without filling your grocery cart with plastic is a process. When you first realize how many items come in cans and plastic, you may feel overwhelmed. Take it one thing at a time, and you can do this.

Tips:

- Moving away from plastic packaging and cans takes time, effort, and sometimes creativity. Start with items you eat most frequently. That's where you'll see the biggest benefit.

- As you run out of staples such as oils and condiments, buy replacements that come in glass.

- When you clean out your fridge, don't feel bad about getting rid of plastic-packaged foods. You don't have to eat something if it isn't good for you.

- Transfer frozen meals to your own non-plastic dishware or bakeware before heating. Frozen food containers are lined in plastic.

- Avoid take-out containers, to-go boxes, and take-out coffee cups. They are often either styrofoam or plastic-lined paper. If you put hot food or hot drinks in them, the chemicals in the containers will leach into your food. Consider carrying silicone bags to use instead of takeout boxes and always bring your own plastic-free thermos to the coffee shop. You might even get a discount.

- Cook more meals from scratch. The more you cook, the more fresh ingredients you'll buy and the fewer packaged foods you'll eat.

- Buy an Instant Pot (or any brand of electric pressure cooker). A lot of common canned foods are quick and easy to make in an Instant Pot. Soups, stews, yams, and carrots can be cooked in minutes. And most importantly, beans! You can go from a bag of rock-hard, dried beans to perfectly-cooked, delicious beans in under an hour. The diet in this book recommends beans every day. If you are also avoiding cans, you have to cook your beans from scratch. You can cook them on the stove, in a slow cooker, or in an Instant Pot. The Instant Pot is by far the easiest and least time-intensive option.

Drink clean water

So long as water is clear, it looks clean. Unfortunately, it's not so simple.

In the United States, all tap water has some degree of chemical contamination. To find out what's in your tap water, you can call your local water authority. Water is regulated under the Environmental Protection Agency and test results are available to the public. You can also enter your zipcode into the Environmental Working Group's tap water database (www.ewg.org/tapwater).

Investigating this can be eye opening. My tap water has arsenic, and my daughter's water in Boulder, CO actually has testosterone in it. Just what a woman with PCOS needs to be drinking—more testosterone!

About 75% of the U.S. population have fluoridated water coming out of the tap. Public utilities began fluoridating water in the 1940s to prevent tooth decay. Today, although there is very little high-quality scientific evidence to support this controversial practice, water fluoridation is extremely widespread. What is clear is that both men and women who are trying to have a baby should not drink fluoride. In men, fluoridated water is toxic to the testes and decreases the amount of sperm they produce. In women, fluoride disrupts reproductive hormones in a way that mimics PCOS, and in fact, a recent study showed that even low levels of fluoride significantly exacerbate PCOS symptoms. Consequently, it's not surprising that in the United States, counties with higher levels of fluoride in their water experience overall decreased fertility.[13,14,15,16,17,18]

In addition to fluoride and industrial contaminants, your tap water likely contains small amounts of chlorine. Water chlorination is one of the greatest health achievements of the 20th century and has been critical to stopping the spread of waterborne diseases such as typhoid. Even today, chlorine kills pathogens such as giardia and e-coli. And that's great. But, by the time chlorine gets to your tap, it's done its job and is now a problem. Chlorine kills all bacteria, and even in small amounts, it is deadly to your gut microbiome. Chlorinated drinking water is linked to gut dysbiosis and colorectal cancer.[19]

Contaminants, particularly lead and copper, can also be introduced into your tap water from your pipes. In the United States, there are literally millions of lead water pipes that need to be replaced, plus millions more that are copper held together with lead solder. Plastic water pipes also seem to contaminate water with a wide array of toxic chemicals. Your water company can tell you what type of municipal pipes your water travels through, but the only way to really know your drinking water is safe is to have the water in your home tested by a state-certified lab.

Now if you think that bottled water is better, think again. For all its problems, tap water is cleaner and more regulated than bottled water. First of all, most bottled water is just filtered municipal water, anyway. But because of the packaging, processing, and looser oversight, bottled water is full of plastic. Literally, the actual water in the bottle is full of microscopic pieces of plastic known as microplastics.

According to a recent study, an American who drinks only bottled water for a year will consume about 90,000 plastic particles. For comparison, drinking tap water "only" adds about 4000 pieces of microplastic to your yearly plastic diet.[20]

Eating and drinking plastic

Plastic contamination of our food and water supply is a monumental problem. For most people, drinking water is the largest known dietary source of microplastics. Shellfish, beer, and salt are the next known largest contributors. "Known" is key here because for most food sources, we don't have data yet. The World Wildlife Federation recently released an incredible resource, yourplasticdiet.org, that is worth exploring.

At the end of the day, there are no perfect solutions, but filtering your tap water is by far the best solution. When you filter your own water, you control the quality of the water you drink. No matter what filtering system you invest in, it is cheaper than bottled water.[21]

The world of water filters is a black hole of options—different sizes, different prices, and different technology. Some filter heavy metals, some don't. Some filter nanoparticles like plastics, some don't. Some filter fluoride, chlorine, and pharmaceuticals, some don't.

If you can afford it and can fit it under your sink, a reverse osmosis water filtration system is the best one to get. It removes high quantities of virtually all types of water contaminants.

Tips:
- Use filtered water for drinking and cooking. If you are going to swallow the water, it should be filtered.

- Never use hot tap water for drinking, cooking, or food prep. Hot water is much more likely to leach contaminants from your pipes and water heater.

- No matter what type of water filter you use, make sure you change the filters according to the manufacturer's recommended schedule.

- If you use a countertop or pitcher water filtration system, make sure you aren't storing your water in a plastic container, even if it says that it is BPA free. Use filtered water right away or transfer it into a glass carafe for storage.

- If your water is very contaminated, even the best home filter system won't make it safe. Be sure to get annual reports from your local water authority. If you are drinking private well water, get it tested. And if there is any chance you have lead pipes, you need to have the water tested in your sink.[22]

- Carry a stainless steel or glass water bottle full of home-filtered water everywhere you go.

- At work or on-the-go, avoid drinking from water coolers that have those big plastic bottles on top. They are full of BPA and microplastics.

- Unless they say they have a filter, most public drinking fountains don't contain water filters. They are just tap water. Even so, when you are out and about, if you need to refill your water bottle, tap water is the way to go.

Week 4 organizer

This week, spend most of your energy on fasting. When you start to feel less hungry and more clear-headed, sometime on Day 3 or 4, tackle your kitchen. Everyone goes about this differently. But by the end of the week, I hope you have a plan in place to dramatically limit the amount of plasticizers and other endocrine disruptors that you eat and drink.

To-do list

- ☐ Inventory all of the plastic in your kitchen.

- ☐ Make a list of items to replace and make a plan for getting it done.

- ☐ Find out what's in your tap water. Call your local water authority. Enter your zipcode at www.ewg.org/tapwater.

- ☐ Buy a stainless steel or glass water bottle.

- ☐ Buy a stainless steel or glass thermos.

- ☐ Replace plastic kitchen items (spatulas, spoons, dishware, drinkware, colander, butter dish...) with non-plastic alternatives.

☐ Invest in glass food storage containers.

☐ Replace plastic appliances with plastic-free alternatives.

☐ Buy an Instant Pot.

☐ Install a water filtration system (reverse osmosis).

Meal planner

* Fill this out on Sunday of Week 3, before the start of Week 4. You may want to plan a fancy Sunday brunch to celebrate the end of your fast.

	Breakfast	**Lunch**	**Dinner**	**Misc**
Mon	ProLon	ProLon	ProLon	ProLon
Tues	ProLon	ProLon	ProLon	ProLon
Wed	ProLon	ProLon	ProLon	ProLon
Thurs	ProLon	ProLon	ProLon	ProLon
Fri	ProLon	ProLon	ProLon	ProLon
Sat				
Sun				

Grocery list

* Buy organic and avoid cans and plastic packaging when possible. Because you are fasting this week, you only need food for your two non-fasting days. If you are not fasting, use the same shopping list from last week.

☐ Greens, enough for two days

☐ Salad stuff, enough for two days

☐ ½ pound of dried beans, any type

☐ Soup, broth or tomato based, not cream based (choose boxes or jars instead of cans, or plan to make your own from scratch), for your first post-fast meals

_____

_____

_____

_____

_____

_____

_____

_____

_____

_____

_____

_____

_____

Daily checklist
* One of the benefits of fasting is a much-simplified checklist.

	M	T	W	Th	F	Sa	Su
Wake up at ____ AM							
ProLon breakfast at ____ AM							
Morning sunshine, 20-30 minutes							
ProLon lunch							
ProLon dinner finishes at ____ PM							
Switch to evening, dim-light mode at ____ PM							
Take melatonin, 1 mg, about 2 hours before bed							
Take melatonin, 2 mg, right at bedtime							
In bed at ____ PM							
Ovulation monitoring							
Sunday prep for next week							

Sunday planner

☐ Take your weekly measurements. See page 325 in the workbook.

☐ Read over Week 5's information.

☐ Plan Week 5's meals on page 138. (See page 331 for ideas.)

☐ Build Week 5's grocery list on page 139.

☐ Go grocery shopping.

CHAPTER 8

Month 2, Week 5

*C*ongratulations! You are one-third of the way through the 12-week Fertility Fast Track, and you have completed one round of the Fasting Mimicking Diet. I hope last week was amazing for you.

Before we jump into this week, I want to remind you of all of the habits that you were working on before your fasting week.

- Establishing an eating window: _____AM to _____PM.
- Eating a bigger breakfast and a smaller dinner.
- Getting 20 to 30 minutes of morning sunshine.
- Eating ½ cup of beans every day.
- Eating a salad with dinner every day.
- Dimming lights in the evening, starting after dinner around __ PM.
- Taking supplements: berberine three times a day before meals plus other supplements at bedtime.
- Taking melatonin: a low dose two hours before bedtime and a higher dose at bedtime.

- Establishing a seven to eight hour sleeping window: _____ PM to _____ AM.
- Monitoring your ovulation.

Phew!

This week, your main goal is to get back into the swing of things. You're already doing a lot! The good news is that this is the backbone of the Fertility Fast Track.

In the next eight weeks, you'll gain weekly habits to help you get some exercise and further improve your diet. You'll learn techniques to lower stress, which is unhealthy for you and your fertility. You'll continue to remove toxic chemicals from your life. And you'll make a few additional small changes that studies show improve fertility in PCOS women. But there are no more enormous schedule shifts.

This week, your goals are to:

1. Start a simple walking program.
2. Replace processed foods with healthier alternatives.

Both of these habits improve female fertility and overall wellness. They take some time and planning, but they are well worth the effort.

Walk 30 minutes every day

Whether you already exercise or the very word, "exercise," makes you break out in hives, you should add 30 minutes of walking to your daily routine.

Fortunately, physical activity can be spread throughout the day so you don't need to do all 30 minutes in one go. Probably the most successful advice I give to patients is, "Go for a 10-minute walk after every meal." It's a relatively easy thing to add to your day, and it gets you 30 minutes of daily movement.

A post-meal walk is particularly healthy for PCOS women because it lowers post-meal blood sugar. After eating, insulin-resistant women like us often experience a blood sugar spike. When your blood sugar goes up, your insulin goes up. This encourages weight gain and aggravates insulin resistance. More than any other activity, gentle walking prevents post-meal blood sugar spikes. A short walk after every meal is a simple way to reduce insulin resistance and thereby reduce the severity of PCOS.[1]

So, it shouldn't be surprising that walking, more than any other type of exercise, increases fertility in all women, and especially in obese women. Women who walk get pregnant faster than women who don't.[2,3]

This week, start walking. If 10 minutes, three times per day doesn't work with your schedule, pick two meals and walk for 15 minutes after each of them. I recommend that you take at least one of your walks after breakfast because then you can combine a morning walk with your morning dose of sunshine. And that's efficient as well as healthy.

Tips:

- Anytime it's possible to walk outside, you should. Going outside several times a day, regardless of the weather, is good for your circadian rhythm. If you only go out for 10 minutes, don't wear sunscreen or sunglasses so you get the full benefit of the sun's rays.

- Wear sensible shoes. If you wear heels to work, throw a pair of flats in your bag.

- There's no right or wrong way to walk. Move at whatever speed is comfortable.

- Sometimes, you just can't get outside. If the weather is terrible or if you are someplace where walking outside isn't safe, then find a way to exercise inside. If your indoor space is large enough, go for an indoor walk. Otherwise, consider using an online program to guide you through a mini yoga class that you can do in your living room. www.doyogawithme.com is a good place to start.

Eat the way your great-grandma ate

It's time to really turn the clock back on your diet. Think about the foods that you eat over the course of a day. Which ones simply didn't exist 200 years ago?

These are highly processed foods, edible items that have been processed in such a way that they no longer deliver the nutrition of natural foods and, instead, contain unnatural ingredients that are bad for you.

Highly processed foods aren't created by chefs in a kitchen; they are created by food engineers in a lab. Natural ingredients, such as fruits and vegetables, are ground up and separated into flavor and texture components. Highly nutritious but less palatable elements, such as fruit skins and rice bran, are discarded. Whatever happens next is a trademark secret of each individual company and product. Some combination of naturally and artificially derived ingredients, plus preservatives, get mixed together and formed into pleasing flavors, textures, shapes, and colors. Food items are packaged in even more pleasing boxes, bags, and cans, and are shipped to grocery stores bearing "use by" dates that may be years in the future. We call these items "food," but I'm not sure that's the right word.

In general, if it didn't exist 200 years ago, it's probably not something you should eat today. Back in the early 1800s, the food people bought looked pretty much the same as it looked when it was harvested. There were fruits and vegetables, meats, cheeses, nuts, and coarse-ground flours. Highly processed foods didn't exist. People didn't eat modern food preservatives, artificial colors, artificial flavors, trans fats, and emulsifiers because they hadn't been invented yet.

People bought ingredients (or grew them) and then cooked them. Foods could be preserved by canning, fermenting, drying, or storing in an ice house. But most food was eaten fresh.

Plastic wrap and cellophane bags didn't exist. Cold breakfast cereal and soda pop hadn't been developed. The machines that would someday turn flour into crackers shaped like tiny fish weren't even a twinkle in an inventor's eye.

Food processing history

I used to tell patients to eat the way people ate 100 years ago, but then I discovered that 100 years wasn't going back far enough. The first artificial food colors and flavors were invented in the 1850s and were widely available (and sometimes killing and maiming people) by the turn of the century. In 1906, the U.S. Congress passed the Pure Food and Drugs Act to outlaw the use of known poisonous substances, such as lead, arsenic, and mercury, as food colorings and to require, for the first time, that products label ingredients as "natural" or "imitation."

I'm not quite sure why we humans love to create and eat fake food, but we do, and we've been doing it for a *long* time.

This is the way you should aspire to eat. Buy food that looks the way it looked when it was harvested. Cook it and eat it.

Processed food is toxic. It harms your health and lowers your fertility. The benefits of eating natural food, the kind that your great-great-great-great grandmothers ate, are enormous.

- Natural foods are more satisfying, so you naturally eat less. Processed foods cause people to eat more and gain more weight. Instead of making you feel full, they actually make you hungrier.[4]

Eating fast food, even just once per week, increases your risk of infertility. Women who eat fast food four times per week have double the rates of infertility compared to women who don't eat fast food.[5]

Sodas (and fruit juices, too) increase your risk of premature death and they lower your chances of getting pregnant. Just one soda per day lowers female fertility by 25%.[6,7]

A diet rich in fruits, vegetables, and plant-based fats and proteins increases longevity and female fertility.[8]

We all know that beans, apples, broccoli, and chicken are healthier than potato chips, burgers, fries, and frozen pizza. So why do we eat junk food?

Western society makes it hard to eat healthy. We are all strapped for time and money. Unfortunately, finding recipes, shopping for ingredients, cooking, and cleaning up afterwards takes considerable time and money. Junk food is fast, easy, cheap, and engineered to be addictively delicious.

The way I look at it, junk food may feel like a good deal in the moment but it is actually extraordinarily expensive; you just pay the price later. Processed foods are full of sugar, salt, fat, and chemical additives, and they lack nutrients and fiber. Half of all Americans have a chronic disease caused by poor diet. Worldwide, about 20% of all deaths every year are caused by eating too much processed food and not enough healthy, nutrient-rich food. Simply put, junk food makes you sick. Being sick is expensive. Additionally, junk food shortens your life. It literally steals years off the end of your lifespan. In the long run, eating junk food will cost you an incredible amount of money and time.[9]

If you want to live a healthy PCOS life and get pregnant, you need to replace processed foods with natural, wholesome, nutrient- and fiber-rich foods. To make this easier, I've collected a list of my favorite meals on page 331. Here are some more ideas to make the move away from processed foods a bit easier.

Tips:

- Learn to identify highly-processed foods in the store so you can avoid them. They always come in packages and contain long lists of ingredients that are hard to read. Sometimes they pretend to be healthy by posting health claims on their boxes. Don't fall for it. If you need to be a chemist to recognize the ingredients, *do not eat it.*

- In restaurants, your best bet is to choose an item that contains a lot of vegetables and isn't fried. That way, you know you are getting nutrients and fiber.

- Keep cooking simple. Find easy recipes that have five ingredients or fewer. The internet is a treasure trove of recipes.

- Make any meal healthier and more substantial by adding a simple fruit or veggie side. Some of my favorites: a slice of melon, steamed carrots, broiled asparagus, a bowl of grapes, or a roasted sweet potato.

- Find cookbooks you like by going to the library and test-driving a whole stack of them. Look for recipes that are veggie heavy and don't rely on prepackaged ingredients such as taco mix or cream of mushroom soup.

Week 5 organizer

Week 5 is all about practicing your habits from last month, starting a new walking routine, and replacing processed foods with healthy, natural, old-fashioned, unprocessed foods.

To-do list

☐ Keep a pair of walking shoes or flats in your work bag so you can take a post-lunch walk.

☐ Check out some cookbooks from your local library or buy some.

Meal planner

* Make as many meals from scratch as possible. Remember that breakfast should be the biggest meal of the day and dinner should be the smallest.

	Breakfast	Lunch	Dinner	Misc
Mon				
Tues				
Wed				
Thurs				
Fri				
Sat				
Sun				

Grocery list

* Buy organic. Avoid cans, plastic packaging, and highly processed foods.

- ☐ Greens, 1 pound carton of prewashed mixed salad greens

- ☐ Salad accessories (veggies, fruits, nuts, dressing)

- ☐ 1 pound of dried beans, any type

_____

_____

_____

_____

_____

_____

_____

_____

_____

_____

_____

_____

_____

_____

_____

_____

_____

_____

Daily checklist

	M	T	W	Th	F	Sa	Su
Eat ½ cup of beans, anytime							
Wake up at _____AM							
Pre-breakfast berberine							
Breakfast at _____AM, biggest meal of the day							
Post-breakfast 10 minute walk							
Morning sunshine, 20-30 minutes							
Pre-lunch berberine			.				
Lunch, medium meal of the day							
Post-lunch 10 minute walk							
Pre-dinner berberine							
Dinner at _____PM, smallest meal of the day							
Dinner salad							
Dinner finishes at _____PM							
Post-dinner 10 minute walk							
Switch to evening, dim-light mode at _____PM							
Take melatonin, 1 mg, about 2 hours before bed							
Supplements							
Take melatonin, 2 mg, right at bedtime							
In bed at _____PM							
Ovulation monitoring							
Sunday prep for next week							

Sunday planner

- ☐ Take your weekly measurements. See page 325 in the workbook.

- ☐ Read over Week 6's information.

- ☐ Order your next ProLon box, if you haven't already.

- ☐ Plan Week 6's meals on page 154. (See page 331 for ideas.)

- ☐ Build Week 6's grocery list on page 155.

- ☐ Go grocery shopping.

CHAPTER 9

Month 2, Week 6

This week, we are going to continue optimizing your diet for enhanced health and fertility. There are two tweaks to your diet and two tweaks to your eating schedule:

1. Increase your half cup of beans to one full cup of beans per day.
2. Eat at least two full cups of fruits, veggies, or other plants with every meal.
3. Shrink your eating window by one hour.
4. Minimize snacking.

Because our bodies are literally built out of the foods we consume, we simply must eat highly nutritious foods if we want a healthy body. Supplements and vitamins can fill in the gaps, but scientists haven't mapped the nutritional content of every type of food and we still don't know what all of these nutrients do. Even if we did, we cannot fit the entirety of human nutrition into a pill.

Most of the nutrients you need come from plants. To be healthy, a person must eat a large quantity and wide variety of fruits, vegetables, nuts, beans, and whole grains. If you are already eating a daily dinner salad and half a cup of beans and if you are replacing processed foods with unprocessed foods, then you are doing great. This week's dietary changes—adding more beans, fruits, and vegetables—won't be a big deal.

Additionally, I will show you how to refine your time-restricted eating schedule. By completing your first round of the fasting mimicking diet, you have trained your body to shift between sugar-burning and fat-burning metabolism, so you shouldn't need to eat as often to feel good. This is a great opportunity to improve your insulin function by reducing the amount of time you spend eating. You can still eat the same quantity of food; just eat it over a smaller window and in fewer sittings. Move dinner forward by another hour to increase your nightly fast to 13 hours. And don't snack between meals.

By the end of this week, you will be a time-restricted eating pro. You will be eating at least six cups of plant-based foods and approximately 30 grams of fiber every day. This is a wonderfully healthy eating plan that will improve every aspect of your health. And, of course, it will support every aspect of your fertility.

Eat one cup of beans per day

As I mentioned back in Week 2 (page 82), beans are one of the healthiest foods you can eat. A diet rich in beans improves blood sugar levels, insulin resistance, cholesterol levels, cardiovascular health, and fertility. Beans are rich in antioxidants that can protect organs throughout the body from oxidative damage. When people include beans in a meal, they tend to feel full afterwards. This satiety lasts for several hours, which reduces snacking and increases weight loss.[1,2,3,4]

One cup of beans or legumes contains about 15 grams of fiber. Humans can't digest fiber so it reaches your intestines intact. The microbes in your gut microbiome *love* fiber. It is their primary source of food. One cup of beans per day keeps the microbes in your intestines happy, healthy, and fed.

On the Fertility Fast Track, you start at half a cup of beans or lentils per day because that gives your digestive tract a chance to get accustomed to them. Some people do feel a little gassy when they add beans to their diet, but after a few weeks, your body adapts and the gassiness goes away.[5]

If you currently feel okay eating half a cup of beans, this week you should increase your bean consumption to one full cup. Check the menu inspirations (page 331) for lots of bean recipe ideas.

Tips:

- When cooking dry beans, one cup of dry beans weighs about half a pound and makes about three cups of cooked beans.

- Per person in your family, cook half a pound of beans on Sunday night and cook just over half a pound on Wednesday night. That will give you enough beans to last the week.

- Freeze cooked beans to use later by spreading them out on a cookie pan in your freezer and then bagging them after they are frozen.

- For a simple way to add one cup of beans to your daily routine, eat half a cup of beans for breakfast, topped with a fried egg, and add another half cup of beans to your dinner salad.

- You can add beans and lentils to almost any dish; just be sure to pick the right legume. The goal is to find flavors and textures that complement each other, not to "hide" beans so you don't taste them.
    - Red, brown, and black beans go great in soups, stews, and chilis.
    - White beans jazz up tomato sauces and Italian dishes.
    - Add soybeans to a variety of Asian dishes.

- Mix red or green lentils into ground meat when you make burgers, tacos, and meatloaf.
- Mix yellow lentils into rice, millet, quinoa, buckwheat, and oatmeal.

Eat two cups of plants at every meal

Unprocessed and minimally processed plants form the backbone of a healthy diet. At breakfast, lunch, and dinner, you should eat at least two cups of plants that are unprocessed enough that they resemble the form they were in when they were harvested.

What counts as "unprocessed enough?"

- Fresh fruit or veggies, any way you like them except deep-fried
- Potatoes, so long as they aren't deep-fried and you eat the skin
- Beans and lentils, any which way
- Whole grains such as quinoa, buckwheat, and steel cut oats
- Nuts, seeds, and crunchy peanut butter
- Popcorn (air-popped, not microwaved, and not the kind from the movie theater covered in fake butter flavor)
- Smoothies, made from fruit and berries, which prevent post-smoothie insulin spikes, blended with plain, full-fat yogurt or coconut cream, not ice cream[6]

Smoothies

I know many people love their breakfast smoothies. On the plus side, you can blend up a variety of fruits and even add some spinach to make a nutrient-rich, portable, refreshing meal. On the downside, it's infinitely better to chew your food than drink it.

Nitric oxide is an essential messenger molecule that protects the health of your circulatory system. It allows your veins and arteries to relax, lowering blood pressure and protecting you from heart attacks and strokes. Nitric oxide is an amazing, absolutely critical molecule.

You produce most of your nitric oxide from nitrates in food, but only if you chew the food. In order to produce nitric oxide, food must be mixed with saliva and oral bacteria. That's the first step. If you skip this step, for example if you drink a fruit smoothie instead of eating pieces of fruit, you don't get nitric oxide.[7]

I think smoothies can have a place in a healthy diet. Just don't go smoothie-crazy. On mornings when you need to take your breakfast with you—and the alternative is a breakfast bar or a bagel—by all means make a fruit smoothie. But if you have the option, eat a broccoli and mushroom scramble with a side of strawberries instead.

What doesn't count? Any food with ingredients that are so processed they no longer resemble their fresh-from-the-field form, and anything that is deep-fried, simply because deep frying is so bad for you. Here are some foods that don't count toward your two cups per meal of plants. You can still eat them, just don't count them as a fruit, veggie, nut, or bean.

- Bread, even if it has seeds stuck to the crust
- Breakfast cereal
- Canned fruit (The fruit skin is removed, which is where many of the fruit's nutrients are. Also, the fruit is often in a sugar syrup, and it's in a can.)
- Crackers
- French fries (Yes, they come from potatoes, but because they are deep-fried, they are simply too unhealthy to count as a vegetable.)

- Granola bars, and most other bars
- Juice
- Potato chips or veggie chips
- White rice

There are healthy versions of many of these foods that really do provide servings of whole, minimally processed plants. Packaged kale chips and muesli cereal come to mind. I've seen crackers that appear to be made entirely of flaxseeds magically held together in the shape of a square. These things exist, but they are usually very expensive. When it comes to convenience food, products always advertise themselves to be healthier and more natural than they really are, so it's just hard to tell. When in doubt, go back to my original rule: If you couldn't eat it 200 years ago, don't eat it today.

To get ideas for plant-based meals, check out the menu inspiration guide (page 331).

Tips:

- Diversify your diet by including two different plant-based foods at every meal. Plant fibers feed your gut microbiome. Diversity of plant fibers leads to diversity of microbes, and a diverse gut microbiome is associated with lower body mass and lower inflammation throughout your body.[8]

- If a fruit or vegetable has an edible peel, eat the peel. It's full of fiber and nutrients.

- Eat a piece of fruit at every meal: an apple, pear, bowl of berries, or slice of melon. This is the fastest, easiest way to add a cup of plants to a meal.

- Pre-cut veggies, such as carrot sticks, celery sticks, and sliced bell peppers, plus a little hummus or guacamole, make a great lunchtime side dish.

- Replace white rice with quinoa, an incredibly healthy whole grain.

- Get a steamer basket for your Instant Pot. You can make perfectly steamed veggies in minutes.

Shrink your eating window by another hour

You are currently fasting for 12 hours every night. The ideal fasting window for most women is 13 hours.

Women who fast for at least 13 hours sleep better, lower their fasting blood sugar, and lower their risk of breast cancer.[9]

I don't recommend that women fast for longer than 14 hours because if you go too long without food every day, you'll trick your body into thinking that there's a famine. In response, your body could shut down reproduction.

Women's bodies have amazing internal mechanisms to ensure survival and promote reproductive success. When energy reserves are low because of a lack of food, the female body inhibits the hypothalamic-pituitary-ovarian axis, the system that regulates rhythmic female hormones and ovulation. This is what happens in women with eating disorders, for example. Nature limits the production of hormones to protect women from becoming pregnant during times of food scarcity, which could seriously threaten the lives of both mother and baby.

You want to find the fasting sweet spot where you get the glucose control and metabolic health that comes from a nightly fast but don't trigger reproductive shutdown. Most of my patients, and especially my PCOS patients, feel best when they fast for 13 hours nightly.

Reproduction under stress

Of course, women do get pregnant during famines, wars, and under all sorts of less-than-ideal circumstances. Not all women are as environmentally sensitive as others, and for many women, the reproductive shutdown isn't absolute. If you have PCOS, your body is reproductively sensitive to stress. This is likely another adaptation of your PCOS foremothers that enabled them to better survive natural and manmade disasters than non-PCOS women.

The best way to add an extra hour to your fast is to eat dinner earlier. If you can't move up dinner, then it's okay to eat breakfast one hour later. Just don't skip breakfast. You need to eat breakfast to drive down morning cortisol. People who don't eat breakfast have dramatically higher rates of cardiovascular disease and are more likely to die from a heart attack or stroke. Push back breakfast if you need to, but don't skip it.[10]

An ideal schedule is breakfast at 7AM and dinner finished by 6PM. Adjust the whole schedule forward or backward to best fit your lifestyle.

Tips:
- Schedule your new eating window.
  Breakfast starts at _____
  Dinner starts at _____
  Dinner ends at _____

- Many people don't get off work in time to start dinner by 5PM and be finished by 6PM. Do what you can to eat dinner absolutely as early as possible, even if it means taking a "lunch break" to eat dinner before the end of your work day.

- Unfortunately, eating your dinner early may not allow you and your partner to consistently eat dinner together. Instead, consider having a big, social breakfast in the morning and sharing after-dinner drinks (sparkling water, tea, or decaf coffee).

- Culturally, dinner tends to be the big social meal of the day, and dinner parties are usually too late for the Fertility Fast Track schedule. If you want to share a meal with friends, consider meeting for brunch or a late afternoon barbecue instead of dinner.

Minimize snacking

Your body does best when it alternates between eating and fasting throughout the day. Eat lovely, satisfying, healthy meals. Between meals, stop eating. You can sip coffee or tea (no milk, no sugar). But don't snack.

Snacking and small, frequent meals became popular because people believed that a constant supply of food would lead to stable blood sugar and would avoid hunger. Unfortunately, the opposite is true.

In a surprising study back in 2012, a group of people alternated between two different dieting schedules. They ate the exact same number of calories with the exact same nutritional profile every day. But some days, the participants ate all of their food spread across 14 tiny meals and some days, they ate all of their food condensed into three meals.

On the days that they ate only three meals, the participants had more stable blood sugar levels throughout the day and generally felt less hungry. In contrast, small, frequent meals actually made participants hungrier and deregulated their blood sugar levels.[11]

Humans aren't cows. We aren't designed to graze. We feel best when we alternate between eating and fasting. So, during the day, eat filling meals that include fruits and vegetables. Make sure your meals have protein and fats, mostly from beans, nuts, and whole grains. Take the time to eat nourishing, substantial meals that keep you full until your next meal. And then you won't need to snack.

Tips:

- My patients frequently tell me that they don't have time to cook breakfast. Yes, breakfast takes longer when you prepare and eat scrambled eggs, cut fruit, and warm beans. But, ultimately, you get that time back because you won't have to think about food again until lunch. Constantly foraging for snacks takes up a surprising amount of time (and money!) and is extremely disruptive to the flow of your day. When my patients switch to eating a real breakfast, they almost all come back and tell me that it saves them time and expense.

- If eating helps you focus, try chewing xylitol gum instead. It's good for your teeth and reduces hunger.

- Make sure you drink a lot. Tea and coffee are ideal because their strong flavor makes them more satisfying. And the liquid keeps your stomach full.

- On those occasions when you need a snack, choose something small, plant-based, and high-fat. Nuts and olives are ideal.

Week 6 organizer

By the end of this week, your diet and eating schedule will be optimized for health and fertility. There are only a few minor dietary tweaks left in the next few weeks.

To-do list

☐   Get xylitol gum to chew instead of snacking.

Meal planner

* Eat a full cup of beans each day and two full cups of plants at every meal.

	Breakfast	Lunch	Dinner	Misc
Mon				
Tues				
Wed				
Thurs				
Fri				
Sat				
Sun				

Grocery list

- [ ] Greens, 1 pound carton of prewashed mixed salad greens

- [ ] Salad accessories (veggies, fruits, nuts, dressing)

- [ ] 2 pounds of dried beans, any type

- [ ] Fruits to be eaten as side dishes (apples, pears, berries, grapes, melons)

- [ ] Cold veggie sides (carrot sticks, cherry tomatoes, olives)

- [ ] Warm veggie sides (potatoes, yams, squash, Brussels sprouts, asparagus, green beans)

_____

_____

_____

_____

_____

_____

_____

_____

_____

_____

_____

_____

Daily checklist

	M	T	W	Th	F	Sa	Su
Eat 1 cup of beans, anytime							
Wake up at ____AM							
Pre-breakfast berberine							
Breakfast at ____AM, biggest meal of the day incl. 2 cups plants							
Post-breakfast 10 minute walk							
Morning sunshine, 20-30 minutes							
Pre-lunch berberine							
Lunch, medium meal of the day incl. 2 cups plants							
Post-lunch 10 minute walk							
Pre-dinner berberine							
Dinner at ____PM, smallest meal of the day incl. 2 cups plants							
Dinner salad							
Dinner finishes at ____PM							
Post-dinner 10 minute walk							
Switch to evening, dim-light mode at ____PM							
Take melatonin, 1 mg, about 2 hours before bed							
Supplements							
Take melatonin, 2 mg, right at bedtime							
In bed at ____PM							
Ovulation monitoring							
Sunday prep for next week							

Sunday planner

- ☐ Take your weekly measurements. See page 325 in the workbook.

- ☐ Read over Week 7's information.

- ☐ Make sure your ProLon box has arrived. Your next fasting week is coming up!

- ☐ Plan Week 7's meals on page 170. (See page 331 for ideas.)

- ☐ Build Week 7's grocery list on page 171.

- ☐ Go grocery shopping.

CHAPTER 10

Month 2, Week 7

$\mathcal{Y}$ou are officially halfway through the Fertility Fast Track program!

In the past month and a half, you have done so much to care for your body. You have eaten nutritious foods and taken healing supplements. You have improved your metabolism and immune system through fasting. You have begun walking. You have reconnected to the 24-hour light-dark rhythms of our planet.

There is one part of your body that we haven't paid much attention to yet—your mind—which is, simply put, an organ required for the normal functioning of your marvelous body.

It's easy to get lost in spiritual discussions of the mind, the soul, and the essence of being human.

I'm a doctor, not a theologist. What I can tell you is that you have a brain. It is a physical organ made up of a wide array of cells. Your brain has blood vessels. It releases and responds to hormones. It is a critical part of your body that plays an essential role in your mental, emotional, and physical well-being.

The mind-body health connection is powerful. Through your nervous system, your brain is physically linked to every organ and cell in your body. You cannot have a fully healthy body without a healthy mind. Numerous studies back this up.

- Social stress increases your risk of cardiovascular disease and reduces life expectancy.[1]
- Chronic depression increases your risk of heart attack and stroke, and on average, shortens your life by over a decade.[2]
- Loneliness is an independent risk factor for all chronic diseases.[3]

Not surprisingly, fertility affects mental health, and mental health affects fertility.

Of course, infertility is inherently stressful. It is often accompanied by intense emotions, relationship stress, and invasive medical procedures. 80% of women who experience infertility experience clinically relevant levels of stress.[4]

Stress is also a strong predictor of infertility. In a groundbreaking study, researchers followed a cohort of couples with no known infertility risks for 12 months, beginning with their very first months of trying to conceive. The women with the highest levels of alpha-amylase, a marker for chronic emotional stress, had an almost 30% reduction in fertility and were twice as likely as non-stressed women to experience long-term infertility.[5]

Mental health matters, especially for women with PCOS, because we are predisposed to stress and mental health problems.

Mood disorders

PCOS is a risk factor for mood disorders. We have five times the rate of anxiety and ten times the rate of depression as non-PCOS women. Alarmingly, women with PCOS are seven times more likely to commit suicide than non-PCOS women.[6,7]

If you ever might harm yourself, call the National Suicide Prevention Lifeline:

1-800-273-8255. Counselors are available 24/7.

Eating disorders are also classified as mood disorders, and women with PCOS have higher rates of binge-eating disorder and bulimia. If you have an eating disorder and you need help getting treatment, call the National Eating Disorders Association: 1-800-931-2237. They are open Monday through Friday during normal business hours, ET.

Your one goal for this week is to:

1. Take care of your emotional health.

I will recommend a number of mind-body therapies that lower stress and improve overall health. Try to incorporate all of them into your daily and weekly routines. While every woman needs to take care of herself emotionally, we PCOS women need to give our emotional lives extra care and attention. It is important for every aspect of our physical health, including fertility.

Take a yoga class

Exercise, in general, is good for emotional health, and yoga is particularly beneficial. I recommend yoga for a number of reasons.[8]

- Yoga is accessible to women of almost all physical fitness abilities.
- It is not weather-dependent.
- Numerous studies show that yoga effectively reduces stress, anxiety, and depression in women of all ages.[9]
- Yoga is better than other forms of exercise at improving insulin sensitivity among PCOS women.[10]
- Yoga helps normalize hormones and improves menstrual regularity.[11]
- Yoga increases the success of fertility treatments and improves pregnancy outcomes.[12]
- Pregnant women can safely practice yoga throughout their pregnancies as long as they work with a yoga teacher who has been specifically trained to teach pregnant women.

Yoga combines movement and mindfulness in a way that is excellent for both physical and emotional health. Like walking, yoga is one of the few forms of exercise that is accessible to almost everyone. If you start yoga now, you can practice it for the rest of your life.

When patients ask me what type of yoga they should do, I tell them to find a class and a teacher they enjoy. Research supports the physical and mental health benefits of all forms of yoga, even your standard gym yoga class. When people take in-person classes, they receive individualized instruction from their teacher and they benefit from the social community, but online yoga classes are also wonderful. Find the class that's best for you. So, as long as you enjoy it, you can't go wrong.[13]

Tips:
- Recreation centers often have affordable yoga classes.

- Many studios offer punch cards that lower the price of classes.

- Many studios offer yoga mats that you can borrow for free. Just be sure to wipe your mat down before returning it.

- Most studios allow students to show up early for some quiet, pre-class meditation and stretching.

- If you have any injuries or concerns, let your yoga instructor know before class. Most instructors are trained to work with a variety of injuries and can help you adjust movements to make them safe and comfortable.

- If a home yoga program makes more sense for you, there are many, many options out there. Some of my patients enjoy doyogawithme. com.

- If you really don't like yoga, pick another form of exercise to do instead. Yoga won't help your mental health if it makes you miserable. I recommend yoga because most people enjoy it, and there is significant research supporting its impact on physical and emotional health. That doesn't mean other forms of exercise aren't beneficial.

- Start with one class per week. Ideally, over time, you want to work up to three classes per week.

Practice guided imagery

Guided imagery is a simple, passive form of mindfulness that is completely foolproof. All you need is a quiet, comfortable space and a guided imagery recording to listen to. Then press play.

I recommend guided imagery over meditation because I've found that my patients are more successful building a guided imagery practice over a meditation practice. It's easier, and for beginners, it's often more enjoyable. If you already practice and enjoy meditation, you don't need to switch. But if you are new to mindfulness, start with guided imagery.

Several studies show that 15 to 30 minutes of daily guided imagery can significantly reduce stress, anxiety, and fatigue in as little as four weeks.[14,15,16]

Mindfulness practice works by changing the physical structure of your brain in ways that reduce stress response and improve emotional regulation.

The amygdala is a part of your brain that initiates stress and anxiety. In PCOS women, the amygdala becomes more active in the presence of testosterone. Because we PCOS women have high levels of testosterone, we have dysfunctional, overactive, highly-sensitive amygdalas that make us vulnerable to chronic stress and anxiety. Mindfulness practices desensitize your amygdala so during stressful experiences, there is less activity in that region of your brain. And when people combine mindfulness with yoga, their amygdalas physically shrink (which is good) and they experience better coping skills, particularly in high stress situations.[17,18,19,20,21]

Brain gray matter is associated with learning, memory, empathy, and emotional regulation; in general, more is better. Women with PCOS, particularly obese women with PCOS, tend to have less gray matter than non-PCOS women. This is similar to the gray matter atrophy seen in patients with chronic depression. Mindfulness stimulates the growth of brain gray matter. Researchers see dramatic results in as little as eight weeks.[22,23]

There are all sorts of guided imagery programs designed to help you get started. You can listen to podcasts, use an app like Headspace, or check out the mindfulness skills on your Alexa.

I personally love and use Health Journeys (www.healthjourneys.com) as a trusted, excellent, affordable source of guided imageries. They make a beautiful series called *Help with Fertility* for women experiencing fertility challenges. It includes affirmations and positive thought patterns that can support you through this process.

Tips:

- Any amount of guided imagery is beneficial. 30 minutes per day is optimal, but even five minutes is meaningful.

- I recommend starting at five minutes per day and working up to 15 to 30 minutes per day.

- Any time is a good time to practice guided imagery, but mornings and evenings are particularly useful. If your days are frequently stressful, morning mindfulness can take the intensity down a notch. If you are struggling with sleep, guided imagery before bed improves sleep quality.

Use aromatherapy in your bedroom

I like aromatherapy because it is a ridiculously simple and effective way to reduce stress. Essentially, aromatherapy is the use of fragrance to moderate emotion and improve health.

Your sense of smell is directly connected to your amygdala, the part of your brain that registers stress and triggers cortisol production. Studies show that you can significantly lower your cortisol level through your sense of smell.[24]

Aromatherapy is so effective that it is popping up all over hospitals—in waiting rooms, surgical wards, and labor and delivery rooms—as a low-cost, low-risk strategy to help patients manage stress, fear, and pain.

When used in the bedroom at night, it lowers cortisol levels and improves sleep.[25]

All you need are a diffuser and essential oils. The essential oils should be pure and highly concentrated; you'll only use a few drops at a time.

For relaxation, my favorite oils are lavender, sweet orange, and bergamot. I recommend Simplers Botanicals brand.

There are a number of different essential oil diffuser options on the market. What's best for you will depend on your budget, your particular space, and the size of your bedroom.

- Atomizing diffusers are the most powerful and also the simplest type of diffuser. Attach a bottle of essential oil directly to the diffuser, set a timer, and you're done.

- Ultrasonic diffusers are reasonably priced and tend to be fairly durable.

- Hydrosols are oil-free naturally scented waters. You can spray them on your clothes during the day and on your pillow at bedtime. You can also keep a spray bottle in the bathroom and spray into the air for a change of scent when needed.

Calming aromas deliver powerful cues to your brain to relax. Because these scents enter your lungs and potentially your bloodstream, it is important that you use only high-quality, organic products.

Do not substitute commercial air fresheners and scented candles. They contain artificial fragrances made in a laboratory, and they release all sorts of toxic chemicals into the air such as phthalates, benzene, and even lead. In some women, artificial fragrances trigger asthma and migraines. Besides, studies show that they don't work to reduce stress and cortisol. You need to get the real thing.[26,27,28,29]

Tips:

- Every diffuser works slightly differently so be sure to follow the directions.

- Experiment with where you place your diffuser and how long you leave it on for. Find the combination that provides a pleasant amount of aroma without becoming overpowering or stifling.

- Be sure to buy organic oils. You don't want to inhale synthetic chemicals.

Try other mind-body wellness practices

I generally support getting massages, acupuncture, or any other type of gentle mind-body treatment. Most of these practices feel amazing, and if you get several treatments, they lower stress, improve mood, relieve pain, and generally make you feel better. Anything that increases physical and emotional wellness is good for your fertility.

In my office, I offer acupuncture and massage. My patients experience success with both, and these services are so popular that the therapists are always busy.

Acupuncture creates physically observable changes in the human body and in people's overall feelings of wellbeing. It improves your immune system, eases pain, and reduces psychological distress. Several studies show that, in couples experiencing infertility, weekly acupuncture sessions improve menstrual regularity, increase pregnancy rates, and reduce the amount of time to conceive. I've been offering acupuncture in my office for 20 years. Treatments done by a licensed acupuncturist are very safe and effective.[30,31,32]

There are now hundreds of different types of massage and they all claim to be good for you. In general, the risks to massage therapy are low; just don't get anything too aggressive. Massage immediately alleviates stress and anxiety. Although a single session doesn't have a significant impact on long-term mental health, an hour-long session once per week for two to three months reduces chronic stress levels.[33,34]

If you enjoy massage but can't get professional massages, partner-massage and self-massage are also beneficial. Start easy and gentle. An internet search on "self massage" brings up countless resources on how to relieve physical tension and emotional stress.

If acupuncture or massage isn't your thing, other relaxation therapies work equally well. It shouldn't be surprising, but we humans respond really well to things that feel good. Get a spa treatment. Hang out in a sauna or jacuzzi. Do something once a week that nurtures your body and makes you feel pampered, relaxed, and self-loved.

Tips:

- Pick a therapy that you feel comfortable with and choose a licensed practitioner with good reviews.

- Learn how to give yourself an amazing shoulder, neck, and scalp massage. This is a good place to start: www.webmd.com/balance/stress-management/features/massage-therapy-stress-relief-much-more

- Exchange massages with your partner. Massage can be a loving way for you and your partner to interact with each others' bodies that doesn't directly have to do with making a baby.

- Use these treatments as a time to connect with your body. No matter what is or isn't happening with your uterus, your body is incredible and deserves to be loved exactly as it is.

Week 7 organizer

I hope that you spend some quality time this week and in the upcoming weeks reconnecting with all the qualities that make your body special and beautiful.

To-do list

- ☐ Buy an aromatherapy diffuser and essential oils (Simplers Botanicals lavender, sweet orange, and bergamot).

- ☐ Find a guided imagery program that you enjoy (Health Journeys).

- ☐ Schedule and attend a yoga class.

- ☐ Schedule and receive acupuncture or a massage.

- ☐ Learn self-massage techniques.

Meal planner

* Remember to eat a full cup of beans each day and two full cups of plants at every meal.

	Breakfast	Lunch	Dinner	Misc
Mon				
Tues				
Wed				
Thurs				
Fri				
Sat				
Sun				

Grocery list

- ☐ Greens, 1 pound carton of prewashed mixed salad greens

- ☐ Salad accessories (veggies, fruits, nuts, dressing)

- ☐ 2 pounds of dried beans, any type

- ☐ Fruits to be eaten as side dishes (apples, pears, berries, grapes, melons)

- ☐ Cold veggie sides (carrot sticks, cherry tomatoes, olives)

- ☐ Warm veggie sides (potatoes, yams, squash, Brussels sprouts, asparagus, green beans)

_____

_____

_____

_____

_____

_____

_____

_____

_____

_____

_____

_____

_____

Daily checklist

	M	T	W	Th	F	Sa	Su
Eat 1 cup of beans, anytime							
15-30 minutes of guided imagery, anytime							
Wake up at ____AM							
Pre-breakfast berberine							
Breakfast at ____AM, biggest meal of the day incl. 2 cups plants							
Post-breakfast 10 minute walk							
Morning sunshine, 20-30 minutes							
Pre-lunch berberine							
Lunch, medium meal of the day incl. 2 cups plants							
Post-lunch 10 minute walk							
Pre-dinner berberine							
Dinner at ____PM, smallest meal of the day incl. 2 cups plants							
Dinner salad							
Dinner finishes at ____PM							
Post-dinner 10 minute walk							
Switch to evening, dim-light mode at ____PM							
Take melatonin, 1 mg, about 2 hours before bed							
Supplements							
Take melatonin, 2 mg, right at bedtime							
In bed at ____PM							
Ovulation monitoring							
Sunday prep for next week							

Sunday planner

☐ Take your weekly measurements. See page 325 in the workbook.

☐ Read over Week 8's information.

☐ Put your five fasting days on your calendar.

☐ Review the information in your ProLon box.

☐ Plan Week 8's meals on page 186. (See page 331 for ideas.)

☐ Build Week 8's grocery list on page 187.

☐ Go grocery shopping (You can either go shopping on Sunday and buy items that will last until you finish your fast or postpone grocery shopping by a few days so your food doesn't go bad).

CHAPTER 11

———

Month 2, Week 8: Fasting

*I*t's fasting week again! Fasting gets easier with practice and the results of repeated fasts are cumulative. Of course everyone is different, but it's reasonable to expect that this fasting week will be easier than your first. At the very least, your body should be much more skilled at transitioning into a fat-burning metabolism. By the end of this second fast, you should see stronger improvements in your metabolic health markers—lower blood pressure, reduced visceral fat, and lower fasting blood glucose.

During your last fasting week, you cleaned out your kitchen. This week, while you fast, your main goal is to:

1. Tackle your bathroom, including your beauty and personal care products.

Bathrooms can be dirty places, and I'm not talking about germs. Most of us have cabinets full of toxic-chemical-laden products that we put on our bodies. It's time to clean up your beauty routine, from your morning shower to your final touch of lipstick.

Get a vinyl-free shower curtain

Replacing your shower curtain (if you have one) is a great place to start. Most shower curtains are made of polyvinyl chloride (known as PVC, or simply as vinyl). In studies, these shower curtains release over 100 chemicals into the air. Phthalates, which make these curtains soft and pliable, are endocrine disruptors that are toxic to female reproductive organs. Other chemicals, such as toluene, ethylbenzene, phenol, methyl isobutyl ketone, xylene, acetophenone, and cumene, are known to cause cancer or be otherwise hazardous to human health.[1,2]

If your shower curtain feels like a sheet of plastic, it is probably made from PVC. Throw it away. If it has an incredible design and this makes you sad, I'm really sorry. Sometimes, the things that are poisoning us are beautiful. You have to look past superficial appearances to see toxic objects for what they really are.

The healthiest shower curtains are made from natural fibers such as cotton or hemp. Both of these options effectively keep water in the tub and off the floor. Because they absorb water, they get heavy, and if you don't dry them after your shower, they can mold. Natural fiber shower curtains are not perfectly practical, but they are 100% safe.

A better alternative for most people is polyester, which has been around for a while and has a robust safety profile. It is a synthetic fabric but has extremely low levels of off-gassing and its components seem to be safe. It's probably what most of your clothes are made of already. It's not a waterproof sheet of plastic, but polyester doesn't absorb much water. Consequently, even when "wet," a polyester shower curtain doesn't get heavy, and it dries quickly so a polyester shower curtain is much less likely to have mold issues.

Most PVC-free shower curtains are made from PE (polyethylene), PEVA (polyethylene vinyl acetate), or EVA (ethylene vinyl acetate). Much more waterproof than polyester, these petrochemical fabrics appear to be safer than PVC. Because there is so little research about these products, it's hard for me to actually recommend them. They are probably safe, or at least safer than PVC, but no one is quite sure yet.

All things considered, I recommend polyester shower curtains. They seem to be the best combination of safe and practical. I have polyester shower curtains in my house and love them. They come in beautiful prints that don't fade, and they do everything a shower curtain is supposed to do—keep water off the bathroom floor without molding or poisoning my family.

Switch to non-toxic beauty products

The average American woman uses 12 personal care products every day that, combined, contain 168 unique ingredients. Through these products, 8% of women are exposed every single day to known or probable human carcinogens, and 4% of women are exposed to known or probable reproductive toxins. Many women have much higher exposures. In 2017, an online makeup store surveyed its customers and discovered that their average customer uses 16 products on just her face every day.[3,4]

Human skin is highly permeable, and many chemicals that we put on our scalps, faces, and bodies, and in our mouths end up in our bloodstream. Are these chemicals safe?

In the United States, beauty products are barely regulated. Makeup and personal care products fall under the umbrella of the Food and Drug Administration (FDA). These oversight powers were established in the 1930s and have not been updated since then. Consequently, they are extremely limited. According the the FDA itself, "Neither the law nor FDA regulations require specific tests to demonstrate the safety of individual products or ingredients. The law also does not require cosmetic companies to share their safety information with FDA."[5]

While the European Union bans the use of thousands of ingredients, the FDA bans nine (nine!) and has some additional regulations around color additives. This means that in the United States, products are sold to consumers with very little safety review.

Many chemicals in lotions, makeup, nail polish, and hair care products travel through your skin and end up in your bloodstream where they act as endocrine disruptors and poisons. Ingredients that are still legal in American products include:

- **Formaldehyde-releasing preservatives:** Formaldehyde is a neurotoxin and causes cancer. On labels, look for formaldehyde, quaternium-15, DMDM hydantoin, imidazolidinyl urea, diazolidinyl urea, polyoxymethylene urea, sodium hydroxymethylglycinate, 2-bromo-2-nitropropane-1,3-diol (bronopol), and glyoxal.

- **Parabens:** Estrogen-mimicking preservatives. Look for methylparaben, propylparaben, butylparaben, and ethylparaben.

- **Phthalates:** Estrogen-mimicking endocrine disruptors frequently used in perfumes and fragrances. You will rarely see phthalates on a label because fragrance ingredients are protected as trade secrets. The best you can do is look for fragrance or parfum.[6]

- **Toluene:** A neurotoxin that damages your brain, kidneys, and liver and can easily cross the placenta. It's found in nail polish and hair dye. Look for toluene, benzene, methylbenzene, and phenylmethane.

- **Triclosan:** An endocrine-disrupting antibacterial. It can be found in soaps, deodorants, and toothpastes.

Additionally, many personal care products are contaminated with industrial byproducts. For example, it's common for talc-containing face powders to be contaminated with asbestos, which can cause cancer.[7]

If this sounds complicated to you, you're not alone; I agree with you. It's extraordinarily difficult to keep track of all the chemicals you're supposed to avoid. Unfortunately, at the end of the day, you, the consumer, have to make sure the products you put on your skin, hair, nails, and face are safe. No one is doing it for you.

There are three strategies that make this easier.

1. **Use food:** The very safest beauty products are organic food products repurposed as cosmetics. The internet is full of recipes for homemade lotions, shampoos, deodorants, and toothpastes. Coconut oil and shea butter are great skin moisturizers and apple cider vinegar is a surprisingly good hair rinse. In general, if something is safe to eat, it is probably safe to rub on your skin or hair. Even so, be careful. Some ingredients like lemon juice and baking soda can irritate or burn your skin.

2. **Buy certified products:** There are a growing number of certifying agencies that will vouch for a product's safety. If you shop online, you can search for these terms. Here are some stamps that are worth looking for:
   - **COSMOS:** European certification; sustainably sourced ingredients, strict limits on ingredient toxicity.
   - **Ecocert:** free of most known dangerous ingredients; biodegradable or natural packaging; at least 50% of ingredients are plant-based.
   - **EWG Verified:** free of all Environmental Working Group's chemicals-of-concern.
   - **MadeSafe:** free of all known ingredients toxic to human health.
   - **NSF Organic Certified:** contains at least 70% organic ingredients.
   - **USDA Certified Organic:** contains at least 95% organic ingredients.

3. **Research:** The largest database for product safety is the Environmental Working Group's Skin Deep database: www.ewg. org/skindeep. Enter products that you use to see their safety profile, and search cosmetics categories to find better alternatives. To further simplify this process, get the EWG's Healthy Living

app for your phone. You can scan products' barcodes to see their safety ratings while you shop.

Organic cosmetics

Why not simply buy "organic" or "all-natural products?" In the United States, these terms are not well-regulated when it comes to beauty and personal care products, and the regulations that do exist are not well-enforced. If you explore Skin Deep, you'll quickly notice that some of the safest products are not organic and some organic and all-natural products are no safer than standard products.[8]

Most organic products are better than most non-organic products, but it's not consistent. The term "natural" is virtually meaningless; natural products usually cost more, but they aren't any safer.

I wish I could just say, "Buy organic." For cosmetics and personal care products, it's not a terrible strategy, but it's not foolproof.

As you go through your bathroom, you'll likely realize that you have a lot of products. Most women do. On top of the products you use daily, there are the ones you received as gifts, the ones you used to use (and might go back to?), and the ones that seemed like a good idea in the store but that you haven't gotten around to using. Here are some tips to make sense of the madness.

Tips:

- Don't waste time or space on old products. Virtually nothing lasts longer than three years. If you can't remember how old something is, toss it. If you haven't used it in six months, throw it away.

- Wash your hands after applying products. This reduces exposure and prevents you from eating residue later in the day.

- Make sure your body lotion is safe. These products can have an array of dangerous ingredients and we often apply lotion all over our bodies after a shower when our skin is most absorptive.

- Look out for sunscreens. The active ingredients in many sunscreens (avobenzone, oxybenzone, octocrylene, and ecamsule) enter the bloodstream at very high levels. Oxybenzone is particularly worrisome. A potent endocrine disruptor, it crosses the placenta in pregnant women and also leaches into breast milk. Instead of chemical sunscreens, choose a mineral sunscreen with zinc oxide.[9,10]

- Prioritize finding a safe lipstick, especially if you wear lipstick regularly. Your lips absorb lipstick into your blood, and on top of that, we eat an awful lot of it. In addition to all the usual toxic chemicals found in cosmetics, lipstick is frequently contaminated with lead. There is no safe amount of lead, and it is especially damaging to fetuses and young children. Because lead is a contaminant, not an ingredient, it doesn't show up on any labels and may not get flagged in the Skin Deep database. You should contact your lipstick company and ask whether their lipstick is lead free. If they tell you that they comply with all laws, this is a canned response that means they don't ensure a lead-free product; throw the lipstick away. Learn more at Safe Cosmetics: www.safecosmetics.org/get-the-facts/regulations/us-laws/lead-in-lipstick

- Of all the products women use, perfume and nail polish are often the most toxic. If these items are an essential part of your beauty routine, prioritize finding safe products.

Clean up your toothpaste and mouthwash routine

Scientists are just beginning to understand the complex interactions of the human oral microbiome. So far, over 700 different oral microbes have been identified. Only a small percentage cause cavities and gum disease. The others maintain ecosystem stability, help digest food, and initiate the production of key metabolites, enzymes, and molecules such as nitric oxide.[11]

Because of our unique hormone levels, women with PCOS have an altered oral microbiome. This puts us at risk for gum and dental diseases. Consequently, good oral hygiene is extra important. Floss, brush twice per day, use a natural non-toxic toothpaste, avoid commercial mouthwash, and visit the dentist twice a year.[12]

Brushing and flossing your teeth twice per day is a cornerstone of healthy oral hygiene. Chemicals can be absorbed through your mouth into your bloodstream, so I recommend that my patients use nontoxic toothpastes. If you are willing to invest some extra time and money, you can find really fabulous toothpastes that fight cavities and gum disease by promoting the growth of beneficial microbes while inhibiting the growth of pathogens.

- **Xylitol toothpaste:** Xylitol is an alcohol sugar that completely disables *Streptococcus mutans*, a key cavity-causing microbe. People who use xylitol at least three times per day have significantly less plaque, fewer cavities, and less gum disease. And xylitol does all of this without disrupting the beneficial oral microbiome.[13,14]

- **Enzyme toothpaste:** Some toothpastes contain enzymes that promote the growth of healthy bacteria and limit the growth of tooth decay-promoting bacteria. In studies, these toothpastes shift the oral microbiome in a healthy direction in as few as 14 days. Zendium and Intelligent are two brands that I'm familiar with.[15]

- **Probiotic toothpaste:** These toothpastes contain healthy bacteria that crowd out disease-causing bacteria. I like PerioBiotic Toothpaste by Designs for Health.[16]

- **Avoid triclosan toothpaste:** Triclosan is a broad spectrum antimicrobial. It is used in toothpaste because it effectively kills cavity-causing microbes. [17]Unfortunately, it kills everything else, so it destroys the health of the oral microbiome. And it is a toxic endocrine disruptor.

Many people add mouthwash to their daily routine because there is evidence that it fights cavities. Unfortunately, most mouthwashes are broad spectrum antimicrobials, so in addition to killing "bad" bacteria, they kill significant numbers of "good" bacteria. In particular, mouthwashes disrupt your ability to produce nitric oxide.[18]

Nitric oxide is a molecular messenger and vasodilator. It keeps blood vessels soft, flexible, and open, and it decreases blood pressure. Your body makes much of its nitric oxide from nitrates in green, leafy vegetables and other foods, such as beets. The process starts in your mouth when you chew your food and mix it with the microbes and enzymes in your saliva. This converts the nitrates into nitrites. Then, in your stomach, your stomach acid converts the nitrites into nitric oxide, which goes straight into your bloodstream and maintains cardiovascular health.

For this process to work, you must have a healthy oral microbiome that can produce all of the enzymes needed to convert nitrates to nitrites. Our human cells can't produce these enzymes.

When people use mouthwash, their capacity to create oral nitrites decreases by 90% and their blood pressure rises. This raises the risk of all metabolic disease. In fact, frequent use of mouthwash is an independent risk factor for developing diabetes.[19,20]

Women with PCOS often have low levels of nitric oxide so we need to maintain our dental health and nitric oxide production pathways. Start with an oral microbiome-friendly toothpaste. Unless you have dental disease, I recommend that you avoid mouthwash. If you need mouthwash, use an alcohol-free xylitol mouthwash. Be sure to visit the dentist every six months.[21]

Tips:

- EWG's Skin Deep online database provides safety information on the ingredients in most common toothpastes and mouthwashes. This is only a partial picture because Skin Deep considers human toxicity but not microbiome toxicity.

- In the afternoon, chew xylitol gum or eat a few xylitol mints. The xylitol disables disease-causing oral microbes, reducing your risk of cavities and gum disease.

Week 8 organizer

Your bathroom should be a refuge, a place in your house dedicated to cleanliness, self-care, and beauty. It should not be a chemistry lab.

This week, while you are fasting, start cleaning toxic chemicals out of your bathroom and your beauty routine.

To-do list

- ☐ Replace your shower curtain with a vinyl-free, PVC-free shower curtain (polyester).

- ☐ Inventory all of the personal care products in your bathroom. Include any additional beauty products that you may keep in your bedroom, purse, car, and workplace.

- ☐ Check the safety of products by searching for them in the EWG's Skin Deep database: www.ewg.org/skindeep.

- ☐ Make a list of items to replace with safer alternatives and make a plan for getting it done.

- ☐ Prioritize lipstick, lotion, sunscreen, nail polish, and toothpaste.

☐ Schedule and attend a yoga class, only if you feel up to it.

☐ Schedule and receive acupuncture or a massage.

Meal planner

* You may want to plan a fancy Sunday brunch to celebrate the end of your fast.

	Breakfast	Lunch	Dinner	Misc
Mon	ProLon	ProLon	ProLon	ProLon
Tues	ProLon	ProLon	ProLon	ProLon
Wed	ProLon	ProLon	ProLon	ProLon
Thurs	ProLon	ProLon	ProLon	ProLon
Fri	ProLon	ProLon	ProLon	ProLon
Sat				
Sun				

Grocery list

* Because you are fasting this week, you only need food for your two non-fasting days. If you are not fasting, use the same shopping list from last week.

☐ Greens, enough for two days

☐ Salad stuff, enough for two days

☐ ½ pound of dried beans, any type

☐ Soup, broth or tomato based, not cream based (choose boxes or jars instead of cans, or plan to make your own from scratch), for your first post-fast meals

_____

_____

_____

_____

_____

_____

_____

_____

_____

_____

_____

_____

_____

_____

_____

Daily checklist

* Here is your much-simplified fasting-week checklist.

	M	T	W	Th	F	Sa	Su
15-30 minutes of guided imagery, anytime							
Wake up at ____AM							
ProLon breakfast at ____AM							
Post-breakfast 10 minute walk							
Morning sunshine, 20-30 minutes							
ProLon lunch							
Post-lunch 10 minute walk							
ProLon dinner finishes at ____PM							
Post-dinner 10 minute walk							
Switch to evening, dim-light mode at ____PM							
Take melatonin, 1 mg, about 2 hours before bed							
Take melatonin, 2 mg, right at bedtime							
In bed at ____PM							
Ovulation monitoring							
Sunday prep for next week							

Sunday planner

☐ Take your weekly measurements. See page 325 in the workbook.

☐ Read over Week 9's information.

☐ Plan Week 9's meals on page 204. (See page 331 for ideas.)

☐ Build Week 9's grocery list on page 205.

☐ Go grocery shopping.

CHAPTER 12

Month 3, Week 9

*Y*ou are now beginning the last month of the 12-week Fertility Fast Track program! Congratulations!

In Integrative Medicine, doctors and patients are partners who work together to create treatment plans that combine evidence-based therapies with the unique values, goals, and life realities of each patient.

In these pages, I hope you are finding a path that works for you. It may or may not be exactly the path that I lay out. That's okay. Every lifestyle modification that you adopt from this protocol is powerfully healing. The more changes you make, the better, but if you can't do everything perfectly (who can?), you should honor your progress.

Each recommendation in this Fertility Fast Track is a gift that you give to your body, yourself, and your family.

This week, we are going to do some dietary fine-tuning. Up until now, my strategy has been to introduce into your diet highly nutritious foods like salads, beans, fruits, and vegetables, hoping that as a side effect, they crowd out less nutritious foods. It stands to reason that if you add six or more cups of plant-based foods to your daily menu, you'll eat fewer unhealthy foods. In the big picture of your diet, this is effective because, ultimately, it is more important to eat highly nutritious foods than to avoid junk food.

Now at the nine-week mark, it's a good moment for a quick self-assessment. Take a look at your Health Metrics Workbook (page 325). On your diet and daily schedule, as they are today, how do you feel? Are you losing weight if you need to? How's your acne? Your mood? Are you menstruating regularly? If everything is excellent, then the program as it is today could be a good long-term maintenance diet and lifestyle plan. If any of your health metrics are not excellent, then you may be sensitive to some of the foods you are still eating.

This week, we will begin the process of removing highly inflammatory foods from your diet. Your goals for this week are to:

1. Remove all added sugars from your diet.
2. Stop drinking alcohol.
3. Limit meat.

Even if you are feeling great, you should continue with the Fertility Fast Track protocol and make these recommended dietary changes for two key reasons:

1. Food sensitivities cause all sorts of weird reactions in our bodies—rashes, joint pain, headaches, asthma, irritable bowel syndrome, and weight gain are just a few. Even if you feel okay right now, you may discover that if you remove an inflammatory food from your diet, you go from feeling okay to feeling amazing.

2. When you have PCOS and are trying to get pregnant, you need all the help you can get. For the next several months, if a food is tied to infertility, don't eat it. I know it's not quite as simple as that, but if you want to give yourself the best chance possible of having a

baby, there are some delicious and convenient foods that may be causing more harm than good.

My hope is that, at this point, you are eating so many healthy foods that you've already reduced the number of unhealthy foods in your diet. So making a few targeted cuts won't be as painful as it would've been a few weeks ago.

Cut out all added sugar

Sugar is delicious. Humans are biologically programmed to love sugar because in prehistoric times, those sweet calories were valuable and rare. Today, simple carbohydrates are neither valuable nor rare.

Complex carbohydrates, the kinds found in unprocessed fruits and vegetables, are fine. Added sugars—cane sugar, high fructose corn syrup, fruit juice concentrate, maple syrup, honey, agave nectar—are the problem. Whether it's white powder, syrup, fruit juice, or a sugar-derived chemical additive, all forms of added sugar cause metabolic dysfunction.

I know no one is confused about whether donuts are healthy; the problem with sugar is that it's everywhere, even in non-dessert foods, and it's much worse for your health than you may realize. It takes very little sugar to change the way your body functions.

At the most basic level, eating sugar raises the level of sugar in your blood, which raises your insulin levels, which over time increases insulin resistance. This sets the stage for diabetes. Because women with PCOS are naturally insulin resistant, sugar is particularly bad for us. In today's western society, women with PCOS have *quadruple* the risk of developing type 2 diabetes compared to non-PCOS women, and we develop it years earlier.[1]

Diabetes isn't the only potential outcome of consuming sugar. Sugar is inflammatory. It changes your gut microbiome in a way that favors obesity. Sugar exacerbates most chronic diseases. It contributes to the development of non-alcoholic fatty liver disease and heart disease. It impacts mental health and is linked to depression, mood disorders, and Alzheimer's disease. Sugar increases your risk of endometrial cancer and not only that, it feeds cancer cells so they grow more quickly.[2,3,4,5,6,7]

And it is toxic to female reproduction. Sugar increases rates of female infertility. Women who eat high-sugar diets have a 92% higher risk of developing ovulatory infertility. Even if you are ovulating, eating sugar can induce infertility.[8]

Added sugars are harder than ever to avoid because sugar is in *everything*! It's in dessert and soda, of course. You can find sugar in peanut butter, crackers, flavored yogurt, breakfast cereal, condiments such as ketchup and BBQ sauce, salad dressing, bread, and tomato sauce. Most beverages are sweetened, and fruit juice, although natural, is as bad as soda for raising blood sugar. If it comes in a package, if it comes from a factory and not a farm, it probably has added sugar. This is just one more reason to avoid packaged, processed foods whenever you can.

Once you figure out how to avoid sugar, you may find that your body rebels. Sugar is an addictive substance. Every time you eat sugar, the reward centers of your brain activate and your body releases dopamine, which makes you feel wonderful. Your body can become dependent on sugar-induced feelings of wellbeing. When people stop eating sugar, they report intense cravings, anxiety, and binge-eating episodes. Withdrawal symptoms can last for two to six weeks, so keep reminding yourself that if you stick with it, your sugar withdrawal will pass.[9]

When you are craving dessert, check the list of approved sweet treats on page 336. My personal favorite is dark chocolate, especially when I can find 90% cacao or higher. Dark chocolate usually has very little sugar. It's decadent, delicious, and full of antioxidants. The flavonoids in cacao protect cardiovascular health. In fact, people who frequently consume dark chocolate have lower rates of cardiovascular disease, and among pregnant women, eating dark chocolate lowers the risk of preeclampsia. So if you get a sugar craving, reach for a few squares of dark chocolate. Enjoy![10,11]

Tips:

- Don't worry about the sugars that occur naturally in fruits and vegetables. In general, it's better to eat more veggies than fruits, but they are all healthy and I don't think it's helpful to get down to that level of nitpicking.

- Check the ingredients on packaged foods. If any sweetener is one of the first three to five ingredients, look for a less sweetened option.

- On food labels, there are over 60 ingredient names for sugar (fructose, sucrose, corn syrup, agave, and fruit juice concentrate are just the tip of the iceberg). In addition to looking at the ingredients, look at how many grams of sugar there are per serving. Four grams of sugar equals about one teaspoon. Anything more than two to three grams is high.

- Don't substitute artificial sweeteners. Studies show that all three of the most common artificial sweeteners—aspartame, sucralose, and saccharin—damage your gut microbiome, creating gut dysbiosis that leads directly to weight gain and insulin resistance. Consequently, people who consume artificial sweeteners gain weight and develop diabetes just like people who eat sugar.[12]

Cut out alcohol

Alcohol can be a touchy subject because, for many women, a beer or a glass of wine is not just any old beverage that can be replaced with water. In our culture, alcohol is often an integral part of a social experience. It is a cue to both yourself and the people around you that you are relaxing and enjoying yourself.

If you are one of the approximately 70% of women in western society who drink alcohol, I have some bad news: You really should stop drinking now. Here's why.

1. **Even just a little alcohol is bad for you.** Maybe you've heard that a glass of red wine protects against heart disease. That tidbit has been heavily promoted by the alcohol industry. The problem is that any small reduction in heart disease is more than offset by a significant rise in liver disease, cancer, and accidents. Worldwide, alcohol is the seventh leading cause of death and disability. There is no amount above zero that is beneficial.[13]

2. **Women with PCOS are poor at metabolizing alcohol and are at greater risk of suffering liver damage.** Women with PCOS have double the risk of developing non-alcoholic fatty liver disease compared to women without PCOS. For all PCOS women at all body weights, even a very small amount of alcohol consumption, even one drink per week, is associated with a dramatic increase in fatty liver disease. And although obesity is a significant risk factor (80% of obese PCOS women have fatty liver), even lean PCOS women can develop fatty liver. If allowed to progress, this disease can lead to liver failure, liver cancer, and either a liver transplant or death.[14,15]

3. **Alcohol dramatically increases hyperandrogenism.** After a single drink, women experience an approximately 20% increase in testosterone. One of the major goals of this Fertility Fast Track program is to get your testosterone levels down to establish healthy fertility. Alcohol undermines that effort.[16]

4. **Alcohol is toxic to your gut microbiome.** Drinking alcohol leads to gut dysbiosis, which causes systemic inflammation. To restore fertility, we have to decrease inflammation.[17,18]

Alcohol works in a variety of ways to lower fertility, and for PCOS women, there's not enough wiggle room to continue drinking. I'm sure you know that once you start trying to get pregnant, you'll need to stop anyway. There's no amount of alcohol shown to be safe for pregnant women.

Cut out alcohol now. You'll be a month ahead of schedule, which is an extra month of lower testosterone, lower inflammation, improved gut and whole-body health, and overall enhanced fertility.

If quitting alcohol is going to be tough for you, find help, even if you don't think of yourself as an alcoholic. You can have an alcohol problem without drinking heavily or getting drunk. If you don't think you can quit cold turkey today, you have a problem, even if it's a mild problem. And you are not alone.

Problem drinking among women is a silent epidemic. Since the early 2000s, alcohol abuse and alcohol dependence have increased by about 85% in American women and similar trends are seen in other western countries. If you need help, discuss your alcohol use with your doctor and develop a treatment plan.[19]

You can also find information and resources at:

- The National Institute on Alcohol Abuse and Alcoholism: www. niaaa.nih.gov/alcohol-health
- Substance Abuse and Mental Health Services Administration: www.samhsa.gov

Tips:
- Avoid places and situations where alcohol features prominently.
- If you go out, be the designated driver. That makes it easier to order a mocktail or other non-alcoholic beverage.
- If you need to wind down in the evening, replace your evening drink with yoga, meditation, an evening walk, journaling, reading, or a warm bath.

Eat less meat

How much meat are you eating these days? For women trying to conceive, I don't support a vegan or vegetarian diet because it is much easier to get all of the nutrients and protein you need when you eat a little meat. But you only need a little. I recommend one small serving of animal protein (about the size of a bar of soap or deck of cards) per day.

Eating meat generally lowers female fertility and replacing meat with vegetable protein (such as beans!) increases female health and fertility.

- Eating animal protein (but not plant protein) raises insulin resistance and increases the risk of diabetes.[20]

- Eating high quantities of meat daily is associated with a 39% increased risk of ovulatory infertility.

- Women who get 5% of their daily calories from vegetable protein instead of animal protein lower their risk of infertility by 50%.[21]

One thing I've learned over the years is that everyone has their own definition of "meat." For some people, it's beef. Others say it's beef and pork, and still others define meat as any food product that comes from an animal.

I approach this semantic question from a medical perspective.

Beef, Pork, and Chicken

When I talk about meat, I'm mostly talking about beef, pork, and chicken—muscle and organ tissue that comes from land animals. There are benefits and downsides to all types of meat, so I don't have a strong opinion on red meat versus white meat. The healthiest meats, regardless of what animal they come from, are organic and pasture raised.

My primary advice is: Eat a variety of meats and choose the leanest cuts available.

Fat isn't evil, but most people get much more than they need. Fat contains and facilitates the absorption of critical fat-soluble vitamins—vitamins A, E, and K. However, too much fat is toxic to your gut microbiome and causes inflammation.[22,23]

Several rodent studies show that high-fat diets cause obesity, dysregulate circadian rhythm, and lead to an altered microbiome. Specifically, dietary fats reshape the gut microbiome into an "obesity microbiome" that is especially good at extracting calories from food.[24,25]

We see an identical pattern in humans. If a person eats a high-fat diet, she will get a dysbiotic, obesity microbiome. At that point, even when she eats healthy foods, she absorbs significantly more calories than someone with a non-obese microbiome and she stores more of those calories as fat.[26]

The best way to convert an obesity microbiome into a lean microbiome is to eat lots of plants and eat less fat, specifically less fat from animals.

When you eat beef, pork, and chicken, choose lean cuts from organic, pasture-raised animals and only eat a little bit:

- Think of meat as an ingredient, flavor, or garnish, not as a main course.

- Choose grass-fed beef. It is much more nutritious than grain-fed beef. It has less fat overall and contains five times as many omega-3s. Grass-fed beef also contains more nutrients and antioxidants. Lamb, mutton, goat, bison, venison and other grazing-animal meats are also great. As with beef, look for grass-fed.[27]

- The white and dark meat of poultry is fine, but don't eat the skin. In addition to chicken, poultry includes other birds, such as turkey, goose, and cornish game hen. Pasture-raised birds are healthier because they have a more natural diet and lifestyle.

- Pork should be eaten with caution. There is some evidence that pork consumption is linked to liver disease and multiple sclerosis, an autoimmune disease. Because PCOS women already carry risks for liver and autoimmune diseases, I think it's a good idea to eat less pork, and make sure any pork you do eat is thoroughly cooked.[28]

- Organ meat is not very popular in the United States, but most types are extremely nutrient-rich. So long as the source animal was organic and pasture-raised, I recommend eating liver, heart, and kidneys once or twice per week.

- Avoid high-fat cuts of meat such as sausage, bacon, ribs, and pork belly.

Seafood

What about seafood? Is seafood meat? No, from a health point of view, seafood is not meat. In fact, couples who consume seafood twice per week are 60% more likely to get pregnant than couples who eat seafood only once per month. In that regard, replacing land animal protein with protein from fish and shellfish is a no-brainer.[29]

The thing that gives me pause is that so much seafood is contaminated with mercury, antibiotics, PCBs, and microplastics. These toxins are not safe for pregnant women. I eat seafood once per month, and I take a daily high-quality omega-3 supplement. I believe that this is a safe compromise. But I can understand if you want to eat seafood more regularly.

The challenge is that there are no seafood certifications that indicate safety for human consumption. In general, here are some fish to avoid and ones to eat instead.

- Avoid large, long-lived carnivorous fish because plastics, heavy metals, and other contaminants bio-accumulate up the food chain. This group of fish includes shark, tuna, swordfish, king mackerel, and Chilean sea bass.

- In general, avoid farmed fish. Some fish farms are clean and sustainable, but many are dirty, overcrowded, and contaminated with pesticides. The fish are kept alive with antibiotics. This group includes Atlantic salmon, catfish, and tilapia.

- Avoid imported farmed fish because some countries have questionable health regulations. Thousands of pounds of fish have been rejected from the United States and Europe due to high pesticide and antibiotic contamination. This includes imported catfish, pangasius (sold as basa, swai, tra, and striped catfish), and imported farmed shrimp.

- Instead, eat fish lower on the food chain such as sardines, anchovies, herring, and mackerel. Wild-caught Alaskan salmon is also a great choice.

- Look for the Marine Stewardship Council (MSC) stamp. Seafood approved by the MSC is wild and fished sustainably.

Eggs

Are eggs meat? This is a very philosophical question. Eggs certainly contain animal protein. However, as with seafood, moderate consumption of eggs improves human health. In a recent study, a group of obese people were put on a one-egg-a-day diet. Compared to the control group that didn't eat eggs, the egg-eating group saw significant improvements in fasting blood glucose and lower insulin resistance. And despite all of the cholesterol fears around eggs, an egg a day did not change their blood cholesterol levels, for better or for worse.[30]

Eggs are nutrient-rich because their primary purpose is to grow a baby bird. They are an excellent source of vitamins B5, B6, B12, and D. They contain folate, lutein, selenium, and, critically, they contain choline. In pregnant women, choline is an essential nutrient that promotes the healthy development of the placenta and supports fetal brain development.[31]

Consequently, my stance is that eggs are not meat. I recommend an egg a day, on average. Studies show that this quantity of egg consumption improves health and longevity.[32]

Dairy

Does dairy count as meat? Healthwise, it's hard to say. Dairy is funny because some studies show that full-fat dairy improves health and fertility and other studies show exactly the opposite.

We know for certain that low-fat dairy is bad for everyone. Women who regularly consume low-fat dairy have higher rates of infertility than women who consume high-fat dairy or no dairy. Ditch the skim milk and low-fat yogurt.

Whole milk and other full-fat dairy products are associated with a number of health benefits—lower risk of diabetes, heart disease, and cancer. And women who consume full-fat dairy seem to have lower rates of infertility.[33]

However, there is extremely limited but somewhat alarming data on dairy and PCOS. We know that dairy is inflammatory, and it's full of cow hormones. In fact, consuming dairy is an independent risk factor for developing PCOS. The more milk, yogurt, and cheese a young girl eats, the more likely it is she will develop PCOS when she becomes a woman.[34]

Dairy also increases sensitivity to testosterone. Dairy is full of growth hormones (to help a baby cow grow into an adult cow) and these hormones sensitize human androgen receptors. For women with PCOS who already have too much testosterone, this isn't exactly helpful. Dairy exacerbates acne, hirsutism, hair loss, and general hormonal imbalance.[35,36]

Looking at all of the research available, it seems that some women do quite well, healthwise, consuming full-fat dairy products. But I am concerned that PCOS women are a subgroup of women for whom dairy is not appropriate.

My basic dairy recommendations are:

- If you don't already eat dairy, don't start.
- If you don't love dairy, remove it from your diet.
- If you do love dairy, limit yourself to one serving per day of full-fat, organic dairy.
- Fermented dairy like yogurt and kefir are best. Butter for cooking is also fine.

Given all of the conflicting data around dairy, I think moderation and caution are the best approaches. If you don't like dairy, don't eat it. If you do like dairy, stick to one serving per day and only buy organic whole milk products.

Week 9 organizer

This week's organizer looks a lot like the organizer from Week 7 before the most recent fast. Hopefully, you are starting to get into the swing of things and this schedule is feeling more and more normal.

To-do list

☐ Get all candy and dessert items out of your house. Check page 336 for approved sweet treats.

☐ Go through your fridge and pantry. Use a permanent marker and put a big 'X' on the labels of foods that need to be replaced with no-added-sugar alternatives. Either replace them immediately, or use them up as quickly as you can and buy no-added-sugar alternatives as needed.

☐ Replace your evening alcoholic drink with yoga, meditation, a walk, journaling, reading, or a warm bath.

☐ Peruse vegetarian cookbooks for some great meat-free entrees and sides. I love grabbing a few from the library to test drive them first. *The Complete Vegetarian Cookbook* by America's Test Kitchen is a great place to start.

☐   Schedule and attend a yoga class.

☐   Schedule and receive acupuncture or a massage.

Meal planner
* Avoid added sugar and limit meat to one small serving per day.

	Breakfast	Lunch	Dinner	Misc
Mon				
Tues				
Wed				
Thurs				
Fri				
Sat				
Sun				

Grocery list

* Check all labels on packaged foods for added sugars.

- ☐ Greens, 1 pound carton of prewashed mixed salad greens

- ☐ Salad accessories (veggies, fruits, nuts, dressing)

- ☐ 2 pounds of dried beans, any type

- ☐ Fruits to be eaten as side dishes (apples, pears, berries, grapes, melons)

- ☐ Cold veggie sides (carrot sticks, cherry tomatoes, olives)

- ☐ Warm veggie sides (potatoes, yams, squash, Brussels sprouts, asparagus, green beans)

- ☐ Dark chocolate (dark chocolate covered almonds, 90% cacao bar, dark chocolate chips)

_____

_____

_____

_____

_____

_____

_____

_____

_____

_____

Daily checklist

	M	T	W	Th	F	Sa	Su
Eat 1 cup of beans, anytime							
15-30 minutes of guided imagery, anytime							
Wake up at _____AM							
Pre-breakfast berberine							
Breakfast at _____AM, biggest meal of the day incl. 2 cups plants							
Post-breakfast 10 minute walk							
Morning sunshine, 20-30 minutes							
Pre-lunch berberine							
Lunch, medium meal of the day incl. 2 cups plants							
Post-lunch 10 minute walk							
Pre-dinner berberine							
Dinner at _____PM, smallest meal of the day incl. 2 cups plants							
Dinner salad							
Dinner finishes at _____PM							
Post-dinner 10 minute walk							
Switch to evening, dim-light mode at _____PM							
Take melatonin, 1 mg, about 2 hours before bed							
Supplements							
Take melatonin, 2 mg, right at bedtime							
In bed at _____PM							
Ovulation monitoring							
Sunday prep for next week							

Sunday planner

☐ Take your weekly measurements. See page 325 in the workbook.

☐ Read over Week 10's information.

☐ Order your next ProLon box, if you haven't already.

☐ Plan Week 10's meals on page 226. (See page 331 for ideas.)

☐ Build Week 10's grocery list on page 227.

☐ Go grocery shopping.

CHAPTER 13

Month 3, Week 10

*O*ne more week of cuts and that's it. I hope removing sugar and alcohol last week wasn't too bad. I know reducing meat consumption can be challenging because it requires a new approach to meal planning. Meat is such an easy and filling food to eat, and it takes time to find equally easy, filling meals that aren't meat-centric. There is always an adjustment period when you remove foods from your diet, so if you are still figuring this out, that's normal.

As we remove more foods, cravings can become a real issue. The most important thing to know about cravings is that they are a short-term problem. In the long run, people on healthier diets actually report fewer cravings. If you are experiencing cravings right now, remind yourself that they will go away if you stick to your new, healthy diet.[1]

Cravings exist in your brain, not your stomach. A craving is an intense desire to eat a particular food or food group. Sometimes, cravings are caused by nutritional deficiencies, but this is rare. People almost always crave sweet, salty, calorie-dense, non-nutritious foods. We crave foods tied to pleasure and pleasurable memories.

Brain images taken with fMRI show that food, pleasure, and reward overlap in the brain. Although cravings are intensified by hunger, they aren't hunger. When a person experiences a food craving, brain activity is primarily in parts of the brain associated with memory, emotion, and reward. These same parts of the brain are associated with addiction, but not hunger. Not surprisingly, people who are on diets or are avoiding "forbidden" foods experience more frequent and intense cravings than non-dieters, often for the specific foods they are avoiding. There is also evidence that activity differences in the brains of obese people cause them to have stronger and more frequent cravings, but we don't know yet if obesity causes these changes or if these brain differences increase the chances of someone becoming obese. The one thing that is clear is that cravings are centered in the brain, not the stomach.[2,3,4]

Cravings are one of the reasons diets so often fail, and they are why I don't like taking foods away from people. But if certain foods are sabotaging your fertility, you need to know. You also need to know how to avoid cravings and how to deal with them when they strike.

Cravings are often triggered by environmental cues such as images and smells that remind you of a food. They can be linked to places, routines, habits, and rituals that once involved a no-longer-eaten food. It's important to anticipate the times and places that are likely to cause a craving and either avoid them or plan for them.

For the next few weeks while you are adapting to your new diet, get lots of sleep and take care of your mental health because cravings are more likely to hit when you feel stressed or tired. Consider starting a project because boredom increases the frequency of cravings. And don't go hungry. Even though cravings aren't hunger, they are intensified by hunger.

Sometimes, cravings strike out of the blue. These unpredictable cravings are likely caused by your gut microbiome. Your gut is connected directly to your brain by something called the vagus nerve. Bacteria in your intestines release hormones and other signaling agents that travel through this nerve and communicate with your brain. Your gut microbiome can use the vagus nerve to induce food cravings.[5]

When you change your diet, you change the food source for your gut microbiome. In the case of the Fertility Fast Track diet, the bacteria that depend on sugary, fatty, and (coming soon) glutenous foods begin to die. Because they don't want to starve, they send food craving signals to your brain to encourage you to eat what they need to survive.

So, if you feel cravings, especially for sugary, fatty, and doughy foods, recognize that these are the dying cries of your bad bacteria. As intense as the cravings may be, if you ignore them, they will go away. As soon as those bacteria are gone, the cravings will be, too.

When faced with a food craving, see if you can beat the craving without eating. Here are some things to try instead:

- **Drink something:** Many times, thirst triggers food cravings. So the very first thing you should do when you start to crave a food is drink eight to twelve ounces of water, tea, or coffee (unsweetened, no milk, of course). Wait 10 minutes and see if you were really just thirsty.

- **Chew xylitol gum:** Chewing gum reduces hunger and cravings, and women who chew gum eat fewer snacks. A bonus is that xylitol gum is good for your teeth.[6]

- **Take a walk:** A change in scenery can change your thought patterns, and exercise causes a decrease in hunger.[7]

- **Do five minutes of guided imagery:** Cravings are often related to stress. In particular, high levels of cortisol, your stress hormone, cause hunger. Studies show that mindfulness decreases rates of binge eating and emotional eating.[8]

In an ideal world, it's optimal to never snack. For most people, that simply isn't realistic. I'm on my feet all day, seeing patients and giving lectures. There are days when I'm so busy I don't notice whether I'm hungry or not. And there are days when I want to snack incessantly. This is especially likely if I didn't get a good night's sleep the night before. Snacking happens. Food cravings happen, and we don't always have the mental energy to fight them. Here's how to snack the right way:

- Eat a high-fat snack containing a small amount of protein. Fat and protein reduce hunger and create feelings of satiety. After people lose weight, those who eat more protein are more successful at maintaining their new weight. I recommend a handful of nuts or olives. If you are really craving something sweet and dessert-like, try a handful of dark chocolate-covered almonds.[9]

- Eat something spicy. Spicy foods contain capsaicin, an active compound from chili peppers that suppresses appetite.[10]

- If you are craving carbs, eat popcorn. This is an especially good snack for nervous eaters and people who snack in order to focus at work. Air popped, butter-free popcorn is sugar free, dairy free, gluten free, and relatively high in fiber. Compared to other snack foods such as potato chips, popcorn is much more satisfying, and because it lowers hunger, people who eat popcorn eat less overall.[11]

- If a craving becomes intense, go eat the food you are craving. It's almost always better to eat the thing you want than to binge-eat something else. When you do give in to a craving, eat the item slowly and savor it.

Over time, you will have fewer, less-intense cravings.

As you go through these last three weeks of the protocol, be kind to yourself and take care of yourself. You may not experience any cravings, but if you do, handle them as best you can. Try not to cheat, but give yourself permission to cheat if you need to. Health is a long road. One day, good or bad, is just one day. Whatever you do, don't give up.

This week, your goals are to:

1. Cut one additional food from your diet—gluten.
2. Limit caffeine.
3. Make a plan for any pharmaceuticals, over-the-counter medicines, tobacco, marijuana, and illegal drugs that you may still use.

For some people, the benefits of these changes will be subtle, and for others, their health will improve dramatically. Gluten causes inflammation and autoimmunity. Caffeine is bad for fertility. All do if you've followed this plan and if your health is in a different place than it was ten weeks ago, now is the time to reexamine any drugs, legal or illegal, that you are taking.

Cut out gluten

Gluten is a protein found in wheat, a variety of other grains, and the products made from those grains, such as pasta, cereal, crackers, bread, and other baked goods. Gluten is often an ingredient in soy sauce, salad dressings, soups, candy bars, french fries, beer, and, well, virtually all processed foods.

The problem with gluten is that many people do not tolerate it well.

If you are experiencing infertility, you may have either celiac disease or non-celiac gluten sensitivity. About 1% of the general population has celiac disease and another approximately 6% have gluten sensitivity; however, the rates may be much higher. Many people with gluten disorders don't get tested because they don't have classic gastrointestinal issues. About one third have diarrhea, but the rest have anemia, headaches, joint pain, rashes, osteoporosis, and menstrual irregularity. Some are seemingly asymptomatic.[12,13]

Celiac disease and gluten sensitivity cause systemic inflammation that can lead to infertility. Studies of women experiencing infertility routinely find higher-than-expected rates of celiac disease. Some estimates are that among women experiencing infertility, rates of celiac disease may be as much as six times higher than in the general population.[14,15]

If you haven't been tested for celiac disease, talk to your doctor about getting tested. But even if the test comes back negative, you should stop eating gluten.

While some people tolerate gluten better than others, gluten is always inflammatory. When you eat gluten, you produce a protein called zonulin. In normal digestion, zonulin is part of the intestinal response to food poisoning. It opens gaps in the intestinal walls to allow more water to enter the intestines and flush dangerous food out of the body as diarrhea.

Gluten triggers this same response. In some people, it is mild and unnoticeable. In others, it causes diarrhea. In everyone, it causes intestinal permeability, sometimes called leaky gut, which leads to systemic inflammation.

To heal your PCOS, we have to heal your inflammation. Gluten is increasing your inflammation. You need to remove gluten to support all of the other work you are doing to get healthy.

Avoiding gluten is tough. Gluten is in several grains, not just wheat. Here are some of the grain products you should avoid:

- Barley
- Bulgur
- Durum
- Farro
- Kamut
- Oats (if not specifically gluten-free)
- Rye
- Semolina
- Spelt
- Triticale
- Wheat
- Wheat germ

Add to that the dozens of ingredients that may contain gluten and it's enough to give a person a headache. I have a few strategies to make eating gluten free simple.

1. Buy mostly unprocessed foods. In the grocery store, you really only have to worry about foods that come in packages with labels. So long as it isn't a gluten grain, fresh food is always gluten free.

2. When you buy packaged food, look for a gluten-free stamp. It's basically impossible to memorize the list of gluten-containing ingredients so I don't try. I just look for the gluten-free label.

3. In restaurants, ask the waitstaff for suggestions. Gluten is often hiding in sauces. Watch out for croutons and breading. And remind your waiter that you don't want a slice of bread, unless, of course, they offer gluten-free bread.

4. Get a gluten-finding app for your phone. I like the Gluten Free Scanner for grocery shopping. Just scan an item's barcode and find out instantly whether the product is gluten free or not.

At first, eating gluten free can feel overwhelming and complicated. But today, gluten-free diets are so common that there are tons of gluten-free products and resources available.

Tips:

- Gluten-free bread and baked goods, so long as they aren't full of artificial ingredients or sugar, are okay. They are pretty expensive, and the taste and texture can be disappointing. I personally prefer to go without. But if you like them, go for it.

- There are many wonderful, healthy grains that you can eat instead of those containing gluten. Quinoa is my favorite. Corn and rice are easy and readily available. Oats are gluten free, but they can be contaminated with gluten so look for a gluten-free symbol on all oat products. There's also amaranth, buckwheat, millet, and sorghum.

- The internet is full of resources for gluten-free baking, shopping, and restaurant-going. www.beyondceliac.org and gluten.org are great places to start.

Limit caffeine

If you rely on a morning cup of coffee or black tea to get you through the day, you can relax and keep drinking your morning hot drink. But if you are drinking caffeine all day long, you need to cut back.

While researchers have not seen any impact of caffeine consumption on time-to-pregnancy (how long it takes a couple to get pregnant, a marker for fertility), there is a significant link between caffeine and miscarriage.

- 100 mg of caffeine (about one 8 ounce cup of coffee) per day increases the risk of miscarriage by 8%.

- 300 mg (three cups of coffee) increases the risk by 37%.

- 600 mg (six cups of coffee) increases the risk of miscarriage by a whopping 232%.[16]

How much caffeine you want to drink is a personal choice. For women who only drink caffeinated beverages on occasion, it's not a bad idea to quit altogether.

If you just drink a single eight-ounce cup of coffee or tea in the morning, it's up to you. You are fine to continue drinking that cup for now and you can decide later if you are comfortable drinking caffeine through pregnancy. The increased risk of miscarriage is small but not zero.

However, if you currently drink a large cup of coffee or tea in the morning or if you have several drinks throughout the day, you should start cutting back. If you reduce your caffeine intake slowly, you can avoid the worst caffeine withdrawal symptoms—headaches, jitters, anxiety, depression, and fatigue. Over the next few weeks, get down to one eight-ounce cup per day.

Tips:

- Make your cup of tea or coffee last all morning by keeping it in a vacuum-insulated stainless steel thermos. It will stay warm longer so you can sip it over several hours.

- Consider brewing your coffee half caff (half caffeinated and half decaffeinated).

- Ask for the caffeine content of drinks at coffee shops. Some large coffee drinks have more than 300 mg of caffeine.

- The amount of caffeine in caffeinated teas varies wildly, even among types of the same tea. Most teas have less caffeine than coffee. On average, a cup of green or white tea will have less than half the amount of caffeine as a cup of coffee.

- Switch to herbal tea in the afternoon.

- Eliminate other sources of caffeine. Sodas, energy drinks, and energy bars are almost always full of sugar and synthetic chemicals, and they can have more than 200 mg of caffeine in a single serving.

Reexamine all of the pharmaceuticals and substances you use

It's been a long time since you did the prep work for the Fertility Fast Track program and it's probably been several weeks since you last saw your doctor. In three weeks, you'll be finished with this 12-week program, and if everything has gone well, you may start trying to get pregnant.

Look back over your test results from your last doctor's visit. Consider scheduling a follow-up appointment for after this program ends to recheck any labs that came back abnormal. This would also be a great opportunity to clarify your plan for trying to conceive. And it's an excellent time to review your whole medical plan.

In particular, if you are still using any prescription pharmaceuticals, OTC medicines, tobacco, marijuana, or illegal drugs, you should discuss with your doctor (or just with yourself, depending on the situation) whether you are ready to wean off of them.

Prescription pharmaceuticals

With some drugs, you take them forever. End of story...unless there's a future medical breakthrough. I have Hashimoto's thyroiditis. My thyroid is damaged and I have to take thyroid replacement medication for the rest of my life. People with type 1 diabetes need to take insulin for their whole lives. If you have a medical condition that is permanent and requires medication, don't even think about weaning off that medication. That's not what I'm talking about.

If you are taking medication for chronic health conditions that can improve—type 2 diabetes, heart disease, depression, insomnia, GERD, and even some autoimmune conditions—you should start thinking about whether that condition is the same as it was when you began this program. If you feel like your medical condition is improving, then at your follow-up appointment with your doctor, discuss retesting and updating your treatment plan.

In general, you should take the least dangerous pharmaceuticals at the lowest doses possible to feel good and stay healthy. For virtually all of my patients, as they adopt a healthier lifestyle, their bodies heal and they need fewer, less-potent drugs.

OTC medications

Over-the-counter medications are still medications. We often get into habits with antacids, antihistamines, laxatives, sleeping pills, and pain killers. No drugs are 100% safe, especially during pregnancy, so if you are taking any medications right now, it's a good time to see if you can take less or wean off them altogether.

Check out the MommyMeds app developed by the Infant Risk Center (www.infantrisk.com). This is a great place to research specific medications and learn what is currently known about their safety profile during pregnancy.

Tobacco

If you are one of the millions of women worldwide who smoke, please try to quit. I'm sure you know this, but smoking is terrible for you. According to the Centers for Disease Control, smoking reduces your life expectancy by at least ten years. However, women who quit before age 40 lower their risk of dying from a smoking-related disease by about 90%.[17]

You should quit smoking for you.

Now that you want to get pregnant, you also need to quit smoking for your future babies. When women smoke during pregnancy, they are more likely to suffer a miscarriage or stillbirth. Babies born to mothers who smoke are often born prematurely and have low birth weight. They have higher rates of birth defects and asthma, and they have triple the risk of dying from Sudden Infant Death Syndrome (SIDS).[18]

Many women smokers switch to e-cigarettes when they get pregnant. In studies, women commonly report that they believe e-cigarettes and vaping are safer than traditional cigarettes. This belief is founded in e-cig marketing, not science.[19]

Research does *not* show vaping to be safe. The nicotine in e-cigarettes is similar to nicotine in regular cigarettes; regardless of where it comes from, nicotine disrupts the healthy development of fetal lung, brain, and other organ tissue. Vape liquids also contain new chemicals, especially flavorings, that haven't been thoroughly tested for safety. Early studies are alarming. One recent study shows that maternal vaping likely increases a baby's risk for facial deformities, including cleft palate and smaller than average faces.[20,21,22]

Talk to your doctor about quitting. Many smoking cessation products are not safe for pregnant women so you need a plan.

- The internet is brimming with how-to-quit-smoking resources. women.smokefree.gov is a great place to start.

- The American Cancer Society has a free quitline: (800) 227-2345. They offer free coaching calls and a variety of other support services.

- Cannabidiol (CBD) is a non-psychoactive, non-addictive component of hemp (marijuana's cousin plant that is legal throughout the United States). Studies show that CBD can lessen addictive cravings and increase the likelihood that someone can quit using tobacco or other addictive drugs. Although I don't recommend hemp or marijuana for pregnant women, I believe that CBD is likely safer than tobacco. Try 1 mg of full spectrum CBD oil held under your tongue for 90 seconds before swallowing. Take every six hours. I recommend Endoca 300 mg CBD oil. One drop has 1 mg of CBD so it is very easy to dose. You can increase the dose by one drop at every dosing until you find the lowest dosage that provides relief from tobacco cravings. At five drops, you can move to the 1500 mg oil and use just one drop (which is equal to five drops of the lower dosing). You can find these products at www. endoca.com. If you prefer to swallow a capsule, I recommend Pure Encapsulations Hemp extract VESIsorb. Take one capsule every morning and evening. Use CBD at the lowest effective dose until you no longer crave nicotine.[23]

For many women, quitting tobacco is not enough. If your partner or family smoke, you will need to minimize your exposure to secondhand smoke. Pregnant women exposed to secondhand smoke experience higher rates of pregnancy loss and preterm birth. Their babies are at greater risk of respiratory problems, learning disabilities, chronic infections, and death from SIDS.

Smoke residue clings to skin, clothing, furniture, curtains, and car upholstery. Called thirdhand smoke, this tobacco film contains dozens of toxic chemicals. There's nicotine, of course, and there's also lead, arsenic, and cyanide. If you touch something covered in this residue, the chemicals absorb through your skin. When pregnant women come in contact with thirdhand smoke, their babies are at increased risk of lung damage. While the baby is developing in its mother's uterus, the chemicals in smoke residue actually change the way the baby's lungs develop.[24,25]

It's important to have strict no smoking policies for your home and car. If anyone in your household smokes, ask them to smoke outside and ask them to wear an overshirt or overcoat that they can remove when they are finished smoking and before they come back inside. Anyone who smokes should wash their hands after smoking. These policies are important for both traditional cigarettes and e-cigarettes. Like tobacco smoke, vaping aerosol is toxic and can settle on clothing and home items to create thirdhand nicotine and toxin exposure.[26]

For the health of you and any future babies, anyone who smokes should follow these rules:

- No smoking inside.
- After smoking, change clothes and wash hands.

While not perfect, these measures can greatly reduce the secondhand and thirdhand smoke exposure of everyone in your household.

Marijuana

Depending on where you live, marijuana may or may not be legal.

In general, I am a great advocate for legal cannabis, and I recommend CBD for a wide range of health conditions.

However, when at all possible, I recommend that women don't use any cannabis products (marijuana, hemp, or CBD) while they are trying to conceive, pregnant, and breastfeeding. Cannabis interacts with a system of signalling agents and receptors throughout your body called the endocannabinoid system (ECS).

The ECS plays an active role in female reproduction. You have endocannabinoid receptors on your ovaries, in your vagina, and in your uterus. These receptors interact with two primary endocannabinoid signalling agents, 2-arachidonoylglycerol (2-AG) and anandamide (AEA).

During the period in a woman's menstrual cycle when implantation is most likely to occur, AEA levels drop dramatically. After successful implantation, AEA stays low until delivery, when AEA rises in tandem with the onset of labor. Throughout this reproductive cycle, improper AEA levels are associated with ectopic pregnancies, miscarriage, and preterm birth.[27,28,29]

All cannabis products interact with the ECS and change the way the ECS functions in ways that scientists don't yet understand.

Early studies on cannabis and pregnancy show mixed results. Some studies indicate an increased risk for preterm birth, an increased risk that babies are born small for gestational age, and an increased risk that babies spend time in the neonatal intensive care unit (NICU). Other studies show minimal or no increased risk. There are also some studies showing that children exposed in utero to marijuana have subtle cognitive and behavioral challenges through elementary school and beyond.[30,31,32]

In the face of this inclusive but potentially alarming data, I recommend that my patients approach cannabis in pregnancy with utmost caution.

If you can quit using marijuana, you absolutely should. If you must use marijuana, use as little as possible. The negative effects are dose-dependent: The more marijuana you use, the more you and your baby are at risk.

I know marijuana use is common and women use it for a variety of reasons. I've had long and thoughtful conversations with women who are using marijuana instead of potent psychiatric or pain medications. Some women get high for fun, which is a judgment-free personal choice when you're not pregnant. Many other women are responsibly self-medicating and rely on marijuana to feel healthy and function properly.

If you use marijuana recreationally, it's time to quit. It may be interfering with your menstrual cycle, your ability to get pregnant, and your ability to carry a pregnancy to term.

If you use marijuana medicinally, here are some things to consider:

- Try switching to CBD full-spectrum hemp oil. Many people get the same benefits from hemp as they do from marijuana, but without the high. We know that in pregnant women, THC (the psychoactive ingredient in marijuana) crosses the placenta. If you are pregnant and get high, your baby gets high, too. If you switch to hemp, your baby still receives the CBD and other cannabinoids, but at least she doesn't get high.

- Avoid smoking or edibles. Smoking of all types, whether it's tobacco or marijuana, decreases the oxygen in your blood. For pregnant women, low blood oxygen leads to fetal growth restriction. I don't recommend vaping as a smoking alternative because there are too many chemicals that don't have a clear safety profile. Edibles make me nervous because when THC is processed in your liver, it gets converted into 11-OH-THC, known as 11-hydroxy-THC, which is more psychoactive and produces a stronger high than regular THC.

- If you can't stop using marijuana, opt for a high-quality sublingual oil or tincture. You can control your dose, so you know exactly how much you are taking. Because most of the THC and other cannabinoids enter your bloodstream directly through the blood vessels in your mouth, fewer get metabolised by your liver and you get a much smaller dose of 11-OH-THC. Look for an organic base oil, full-spectrum hemp product made by CO_2 extraction.

- Abstain from marijuana during your peak fertility window, and your partner should abstain, too. Studies indicate that sperm exposed to THC behave abnormally. They swim too fast too soon, and are less likely to reach the woman's egg. Sperm can be exposed to THC if the man uses marijuana, but they can also be exposed through a woman's reproductive fluids if she has used marijuana.[33]

- If you live in a place where marijuana is illegal, learn about your hospital's rules for drug testing mothers and infants at delivery. If you produce a positive drug test, will you be reported to Child Protective Services (CPS)?

When it comes to marijuana, hemp, and CBD, only take what you need, and if you can quit, you should.

Illegal drugs and controlled substances

If you use illegal drugs or are dependent or addicted to controlled substances, such as opioids, please discuss this with your doctor and make a plan to quit. Drugs and pregnancy are a bad combo. If you need additional resources, start with the Substance Abuse and Mental Health Services Administration (SAMHSA) helpline: 1(800) 662-4357. They provide free, confidential, 24-hour-a-day information and referrals to local support resources.

Week 10 organizer

Here's your organizer for Week 10. There are no new habits or routines, but if you normally drink a lot of coffee or eat a lot of pasta or bread, this week could still be pretty challenging. Take it day by day.

To-do list

☐ Download the Gluten Free Scanner app to your phone. Scan all of the packaged food in your kitchen, including sauces and condiments.

☐ Clean all gluten-containing products out of your kitchen.

☐ Consider using CBD to help break any addictions you may have. (Endoca 300mg or 1500 mg CBD oil *or* Pure Encapsulations Hemp extract VESIsorb)

☐ Make a follow-up appointment with your doctor for after the end of the 12-week program.

1. Retake any lab tests from your last appointment that came back abnormal.
2. Review all medications and drugs you are taking and see which ones you can wean off of.
3. Discuss your trying-to-get-pregnant plan.

☐ Schedule and attend a yoga class.

☐ Schedule and receive acupuncture or a massage.

Meal planner

* Avoid added sugar and gluten. Per day, limit caffeine to one drink and limit meat to one small serving.

	Breakfast	**Lunch**	**Dinner**	**Misc**
Mon				
Tues				
Wed				
Thurs				
Fri				
Sat				
Sun				

Grocery list

* Check all labels on packaged foods for added sugar and gluten

- ☐ Greens, 1 pound carton of prewashed mixed salad greens

- ☐ Salad accessories (veggies, fruits, nuts, dressing)

- ☐ 2 pounds of dried beans, any type

- ☐ Fruits to be eaten as side dishes (apples, pears, berries, grapes, melons)

- ☐ Cold veggie sides (carrot sticks, cherry tomatoes, olives)

- ☐ Warm veggie sides (potatoes, yams, squash, Brussels sprouts, asparagus, green beans)

- ☐ Dark chocolate (dark chocolate covered almonds, 90% cacao bar, dark chocolate chips)

_____

_____

_____

_____

_____

_____

_____

_____

_____

_____

_____

Daily checklist

	M	T	W	Th	F	Sa	Su
Eat 1 cup of beans, anytime							
15-30 minutes of guided imagery, anytime							
Wake up at ____AM							
Pre-breakfast berberine							
Breakfast at ____AM, biggest meal of the day incl. 2 cups plants							
Post-breakfast 10 minute walk							
Morning sunshine, 20-30 minutes							
Pre-lunch berberine							
Lunch, medium meal of the day incl. 2 cups plants							
Post-lunch 10 minute walk							
Pre-dinner berberine							
Dinner at ____PM, incl. 2 cups plants							
Dinner salad							
Dinner at ____PM, smallest meal of the day incl. 2 cups plants							
Post-dinner 10 minute walk							
Switch to evening, dim-light mode at ____PM							
Take melatonin, 1 mg, about 2 hours before bed							
Supplements							
Take melatonin, 2 mg, right at bedtime							
In bed at ____PM							
Ovulation monitoring							
Sunday prep for next week							

Sunday planner

☐ Take your weekly measurements. See page 325 in the workbook.

☐ Read over Week 11's information.

☐ Make sure your ProLon box has arrived. Your next fasting week is coming up!

☐ Plan Week 11's meals on page 244. (See page 331 for ideas.)

☐ Build Week 11's grocery list on page 245.

☐ Go grocery shopping.

CHAPTER 14

Month 3, Week 11

$\mathscr{T}$he last two weeks were almost all about removing foods from your diet. I'm sorry!

I hate telling people not to do things. That's why I waited to do so until the last month of the protocol. But honestly, as a doctor, I'd rather tell you to cut out sugar, alcohol, and gluten, drink less caffeine, and eat less meat than prescribe powerful pharmaceuticals, surgery, or other invasive procedures. In the grand scheme of things, dietary changes aren't too bad.

Even so, I'm glad we are done and can move on to better things.

Your only goal for this week is to:

1. Experiment and fine-tune this Fertility Fast Track protocol to best meet your unique needs.

I'm going to show you several little additions to your diet and routine that can be extremely helpful. Of course, it would be amazing if you could do all of them, but that's probably not realistic. Even the most devoted health-followers have limits, and if you're not there right now, you're probably close.

Review these recommendations and pick the ones that best address your remaining challenges. This is your week to figure out how to make this program work specifically for you.

Add these foods and drinks to your diet

As I said way back in the beginning of this book, food is medicine. Some foods are especially powerful. Here are a few that I recommend for PCOS and fertility.

Beetroot juice

Beetroot juice is simply juice made from beets. It is rich in nitrates that your body converts to nitric oxide, a potent vasodilator, meaning it relaxes blood vessels and lowers blood pressure. Consequently, it is a natural treatment for hypertension. Studies show that it may be helpful in lowering the risk for preeclampsia, dangerously high blood pressure during pregnancy. It also plays a role in the growth and formation of a healthy placenta.[1,2]

I recommend beetroot juice for all PCOS women attempting to get pregnant, and I especially recommend it for anyone with a history of high blood pressure or cardiovascular disease.

Note that your body can only make nitric oxide if you have a healthy mouth microbiome, so it's important that you don't use commercial mouthwash or antibacterial toothpaste.

Beetroot juice is a really simple thing to add to your diet. You can buy it in most grocery stores (it might be called beet juice), all health and fitness stores, and online.

The standard dosage is 70 mL once per day. This is approximately one-third of a cup or two full shot glasses. It's best to drink beetroot juice at breakfast when your insulin is most sensitive because of its sugar content.

Fermented foods

Fermentation is an ancient form of food processing that employs bacteria or yeast to convert sugars to lactic acid. Historically used to preserve foods before the invention of refrigeration, fermentation increases foods' nutritional quality and, importantly, its beneficial microbe population. Much more potent than probiotics in a pill, fermented foods are alive with trillions of bacteria that can survive the journey through your digestive tract and improve the health of your gut microbiome.[3]

A healthy gut microbiome improves all PCOS symptoms—hormonal imbalances, metabolism, and mood disorders. And in pregnancy, a healthy gut microbiome is critical for a healthy pregnancy and healthy baby. Gut dysbiosis in the mother increases the risk of preterm delivery and infant neurodevelopmental disorders.[4,5]

Consequently, in addition to taking a daily probiotic, I recommend that everyone eat one-quarter cup of fermented veggies every day. I especially recommend this for anyone who is overweight or pregnant.

Personally, I find the easiest way to get my daily fermented veggies is to pack a small container of sauerkraut or kimchi everyday for lunch. If you eat dairy, unsweetened whole milk yogurt and kefir also contain probiotic bacteria.

When buying fermented foods, look for products that are still alive. These can be hard to find because live, fermented foods release bubbles and constantly expand. Left on a shelf in a jar for long enough, they explode. So, most companies heat pasteurize them, preserving the taste but killing the microbes, which means no explosions and no bacteria.

Your best bet is to check your grocery store's refrigerated section (that's where my local shop keeps a few varieties of live sauerkraut) or try a local health food store or farmer's market. If you are interested in making your own, *Fermented* Vegetables by Kirsten and Christopher Shockey is a great resource.

Soy

Soy is a super food that protects women from some of the negative effects of BPA.

BPA is terrible for female fertility and especially bad for women with PCOS. Most women with PCOS have high levels of BPA in their bodies, and high BPA causes elevated testosterone levels, metabolic disease, and infertility.

In a recent study, women undergoing IVF were tested for BPA. Those with high levels of BPA had much lower chances of getting pregnant and successfully delivering a live baby. However, there was a huge exception. Among women who regularly consumed soy, BPA had no influence on IVF success. The soy protected them from the negative fertility effects of BPA.[6]

I recommend that all PCOS women add organic soy to their diets. This is especially important for pregnant women and for women trying to get pregnant, whether naturally or through any form of assisted reproductive technology.

Eat a full serving of soy, such as tofu, tempeh, and edamame, three to four times per week. Mix tofu or tempeh into scrambled eggs. Add it to curries and stir-fries. I keep frozen organic soybeans on hand because I can quickly defrost them and throw them on a salad. I also like to marinate and grill tofu or tempeh instead of meat.

Spearmint tea

Elevated testosterone lowers your fertility. For pregnant women, high testosterone increases the risk of future metabolic disease for your growing baby, and if your baby is a girl, high testosterone in your body increases her risk of someday developing PCOS herself.

There are very few safe and effective ways to lower testosterone. Spearmint tea is one of them.

Spearmint tea is a potent anti-androgen. In studies, women who drink two cups of spearmint tea per day lower their free testosterone levels and reduce signs of hyperandrogenism, such as hirsutism and acne.[7,8]

I recommend two cups per day of spearmint tea for anyone struggling with acne, facial hair growth, or scalp hair loss. And I definitely recommend two cups per day for all PCOS women throughout the pregnancy process.

Be aware that most mint tea in the grocery store is a blend of mints. You want pure spearmint tea. I buy Traditional Medicinals Organic Spearmint Herbal Tea in the health section of my local grocery store.

Try these circadian rhythm tips

If you are having any challenges with sleep or appetite regulation, here are tips to further strengthen your circadian rhythm.

Wake with a dawn simulator

If you want a natural, healthy kickstart to your day, wake up with the sunrise.

When researchers expose people to the growing lights and colors of the sunrise, they see a 50% drop in mood disorders, an increase in morning alertness, and a phase advance of circadian rhythm. This means that people have fewer depression and anxiety symptoms. In the evening, they fall asleep earlier, and they generally sleep better and longer. They feel good when they wake up in the morning.[9,10,11]

Sunrise doesn't always happen at a convenient time. Fortunately, you don't actually need to "watch" the sunrise to get these benefits.

When researchers perform these studies, they expose subjects to a dawn simulator, a light that mimics sunrise, during the 30 minutes before they wake up. Subjects experience the dawn simulator while they are still asleep because our bodies are supposed to experience the sunrise through still-closed, still-sleeping eyelids.[12]

A dawn simulator is an alarm clock-type device that will simulate sunrise for 30 minutes, starting at whatever time you choose. Purchase one that produces a nice, diffuse, bright light. I love my Philips Wake-up Light and keep it on my night table.

Get afternoon sunlight

Any day that you can, sometime around lunch, get out into the sunshine— no sunglasses, no sunscreen, with as much skin showing as weather and propriety allow.

Of course, exposure to sunshine is a balancing act. We all know that too much sunshine causes sunburns, wrinkles, and skin cancer. But the right amount of midday sunshine is excellent for your health.

Daytime sunlight leads to stronger circadian rhythms, more nighttime melatonin production, and better immune system function. Daytime sunshine helps your body produce vitamin D, the so-called "sunshine vitamin," which among other things is a powerful anti-inflammatory. Additionally, sunshine causes your skin to release nitric oxide, that hugely beneficial signaling molecule that decreases blood pressure and improves the flexibility of your blood vessels.[13,14,15,16,17]

These benefits help explain why female fertility is generally higher in the summer than in the winter. Because women with darker skin are more likely to be vitamin D deficient, this summer-winter fertility pattern is especially strong in women of African descent. Women with PCOS are also typically vitamin D deficient, so it's safe to assume that the same pattern holds true for all PCOS women, regardless of their skin color.[18,19]

The right amount of sunshine is fabulous for your health and fertility. Exactly how much that is depends on your skin tone, where you live, the time of year, and even your age.

Here's my rule of thumb: Get as much as you can without turning pink.

In the summer, I recommend that people go outside for 10 to 20 minutes around 11AM or 2PM to avoid the brightest part of the day when you are more likely to burn. But in the winter, aim for the sunniest time and go for as long as you can, up to two hours. If your skin is darker, you need more sun and if your skin is extremely fair, you need less. Additionally, you lose 30% of your ability to make vitamin D from sunshine as you age, so older women need more time in the sun to get the same results as younger women.[20,21]

Hopefully, you are taking a post-lunch walk. This is a great way to get some sunshine and simultaneously improve blood sugar levels. Also consider eating lunch outside or working outside whenever possible.

Watch the sunset

Just as the colors of dawn get you going in the morning, the colors of the sunset wind you down in the evening. So, watch the sunset. The warm colors of the sunset—the oranges, reds, and yellows—program your brain to prepare for evening and sleep.

Receptors in your eyes are highly sensitive to the color of light. When they are exposed to daytime light, which you see as blue light, these receptors convey that information to your master clock, which blocks the production of melatonin. But in the evening, when the intensity of blue decreases and the color of the light warms, the receptors in your eyes cue your body to start producing melatonin again.

This initiates dim light melatonin onset, a critical part of the evening when your body begins producing melatonin and transitioning from daytime metabolism to nighttime metabolism.

If you miss your dim light melatonin onset, your entire sleep cycle gets delayed. Sunset is the best way to trigger this key phase of your circadian rhythm.

So, take a little time out of your day to enjoy one of Mother Nature's daily miracles, the beauty of the sunset.

Add evening light

Most women with PCOS have Delayed Sleep Phase Syndrome (DSPS). This is when your circadian rhythm is shifted later and you are a night owl. But a minority of women have Advanced Sleep Phase Syndrome (ASPS). These reluctant early birds wake up early, before 6AM, and simply can't fall back asleep, even though they are still tired.

If you think you have ASPS, you should follow all of the light-dark advice in this book *and* do one more thing: In the evening, add another dose of bright light to push back your melatonin onset time.

Now, here's the thing about evening light treatments. Unlike morning light, which is pretty impossible to overdose on, evening light therapy is very dose and time dependent. I recommend that you work with a trusted sleep medicine specialist and use a light therapy lamp so you can control your dose.

You should begin your evening light therapy at the same time every day. I recommend starting around 7PM with five minutes of 10,000 lux light. Go to bed at the same time as usual and see what time you wake up. Do this every day for a few days and then assess.

If you are falling asleep okay and want to sleep longer, add another five minutes of evening light. Keep adding light in five minute increments until you are waking up at a time that works for you.

Drink herbal tea at night

If you have trouble falling asleep at night, try drinking a relaxing cup of tea an hour or two before bed. There are several types of tea that reduce stress and anxiety and induce sleepiness. I particularly like chamomile, passionflower, and lemon balm. Chamomile and passionflower are mild sedatives, so they will help you fall asleep faster.

Get more exercise

How's your exercise routine going? If you are struggling to maintain a regular exercise schedule, you're not alone. It's hard to prioritize exercise. Here are some tips for transforming intention into action.

Wear a fitness tracker

One powerful way to increase your daily movement is to wear an electronic fitness tracker. When people start a new exercise routine and wear a Fitbit, they move more than people who wear a simple pedometer or no tracking device.[22]

Of course, it doesn't need to be a Fitbit. Any fitness tracker is great. If you already have an iPhone, the Apple Watch tracks your exercise routines and also reminds you to get up and move at least once per hour.

Find a fitness tracker that works for you.

Do more yoga

If you are feeling okay about your weekly yoga class, see if you can increase to two or three classes per week. An optimal fertility exercise program is:

- Walk for 30 minutes every day.
- Yoga three times per week.

Try an online exercise program

If you need to give your exercise routine a boost, the internet can be a great resource. In general, when people start an exercise program, they begin with enthusiasm but their compliance rapidly declines over time. Most online exercise programs follow this same trend, unless they involve a social component.

I usually advise patients to start with online videos like the ones on Do Yoga With Me (www.doyogawithme.com) because they are the most flexible and are free to get started. Some patients do great with these self-directed exercise programs, but some women tell me that when they work out in their living rooms, they lose motivation.

If this is you, instead of following along with prerecorded exercise classes, try signing up for virtual exercise classes. These are online classes taught by a live instructor. You have to pay for them and they are less flexible because they are live. But, they are much more fun, social, and rewarding. I recommend Gixmo (www.gixo.com) because they offer short classes all day long.

If you enjoy friendly competition, explore virtual fitness challenges. You pick a goal (for example, walking 20 miles), and then you work towards that goal over time, adding miles as you walk them, whenever you walk them, until you reach your goal. I like the yes.fit community and app because they have fun beginner races, such as the Cinderella race.

Consider a few more supplements

Depending on how you are feeling, you may want to consider taking a few more supplements. It probably feels like I've recommended a ton of supplements already, but I'm actually holding back. Really! Here are a few more supplements you may want to add to your daily routine.

Nitric oxide

I've mentioned nitric oxide several times already; it's a molecular messenger and vasodilator. It keeps blood vessels soft, flexible, and open, and it decreases blood pressure.[23]

You can get it from eating nitrate-rich veggies, drinking beetroot juice, and spending time in the sun with bare skin. There are also nitric oxide supplements that increase your body's production of nitric oxide.

I encourage all of my PCOS patients with high blood pressure or cardiovascular disease to take Pure Encapsulations Nitric Oxide Ultra or HumanN Neo40. Take either supplement twice daily, 20 minutes before a meal.

Resveratrol

Found in grape skins and red wine, resveratrol is a powerful antioxidant that is particularly useful for PCOS women trying to get pregnant.

In PCOS women, resveratrol lowers testosterone and decreases insulin resistance. In a recent study, PCOS women who took 1500 mg of resveratrol daily for three months experienced a 23% reduction in testosterone and a 31% decrease in fasting insulin.[24]

It also improves egg quality, especially for women with endometriosis.[25]

For most PCOS women on the Fertility Fast Track program, the core supplements are enough to lower testosterone and insulin resistance, and I try not to overwhelm people with crazy amounts of supplements. However, if you are not losing weight or if you still have significant hyperandrogenism (acne, hirsutism, hair loss), then it might be time to add resveratrol into the protocol. I also recommend resveratrol for women over 35 or those with diminished ovarian reserve.

I usually give my patients Pure Encapsulations Resveratrol, which has 40 mg per capsule.

Ubiquinol

If you are older than 35, if you've had one or more miscarriages, or if you've been told that you have diminished ovarian reserve, you should consider taking ubiquinol.

Ubiquinol is the active form of CoQ10. Most commercial CoQ10 supplements are ubiquinone, which isn't absorbed as well as ubiquinol.[26]

This supplement is a powerful antioxidant that plays a critical role in cell energy production. As we age, our bodies produce less ubiquinol, and that deficiency plays a role in decreased egg quality in women over 35. Several studies have shown that ubiquinol supplements can improve egg viability and reduce chromosomal abnormalities.[27,28,29]

I usually give my patients Pure Encapsulations Ubiquinol-QH 100 mg and recommend that they take two 100 mg capsule three times per day (600 mg per day total). Take it at the same time you take the berberine.

Week 11 organizer

Consider where you are, honestly, in your health and fertility journey. Add as many of the recommendations from this week as you can, prioritizing the ones that address any lingering challenges you face.

To-do list

☐ Exchange your alarm clock for a dawn simulator (Philips Wake-up Light).

☐ Start wearing a fitness tracker (Fitbit or Apple Watch).

☐ Try an online exercise program (Do Yoga With Me (www.doyogawithme.com) or Gixmo (www.gixo.com)).

☐ Register for an online fitness challenge (yes.fit).

☐ Buy additional supplements:

    ☐ Nitric oxide supplement (Pure Encapsulations Nitric Oxide Ultra or HumanN Neo40)

    ☐ Resveratrol (Pure Encapsulations Resveratrol)

    ☐ Ubiquinol (Pure Encapsulations Ubiquinol-QH 100 mg)

☐   Schedule and attend one to three yoga classes.

☐   Schedule and receive acupuncture or a massage.

Meal planner

* Avoid added sugar and gluten. Per day, limit caffeine to one drink and limit meat to one small serving. Eat a quarter-cup of fermented foods once a day, and include soy three to four times per week.

	Breakfast	Lunch	Dinner	Misc
Mon				
Tues				
Wed				
Thurs				
Fri				
Sat				
Sun				

Grocery list

* Check all labels on packaged foods for added sugar and gluten.

- ☐ Greens, 1 pound carton of prewashed mixed salad greens

- ☐ Salad accessories (veggies, fruits, nuts, dressing)

- ☐ 2 pounds of dried beans, any type

- ☐ Fruits to be eaten as side dishes (apples, pears, berries, grapes, melons)

- ☐ Cold veggie sides (carrot sticks, cherry tomatoes, olives)

- ☐ Warm veggie sides (potatoes, yams, squash, Brussels sprouts, asparagus, green beans)

- ☐ Dark chocolate (dark chocolate covered almonds, 90% cacao bar, dark chocolate chips)

- ☐ Beetroot juice

- ☐ Fermented foods (sauerkraut and kimchi; if you eat dairy, also plain whole milk yogurt and kefir)

- ☐ Soy (tofu, tempeh, edamame)

- ☐ Spearmint tea

_____

_____

_____

_____

_____

_____

_____

Daily checklist

	M	T	W	Th	F	Sa	Su
Eat 1 cup of beans, anytime							
Eat ¼ cup of fermented veggies, anytime							
Drink 2 cups of spearmint tea, anytime							
15-30 min. of guided imagery, anytime							
Wake up at ____AM							
Pre-breakfast berberine, ubiquinol, and nitric oxide							
Breakfast at ____AM, incl. 2 cups plants and 70 mL beetroot juice							
Post-breakfast 10 min. walk							
Morning sunshine, 20-30 min.							
Pre-lunch berberine, ubiquinol, and nitric oxide							
Lunch, incl. 2 cups plants							
Post-lunch 10 min. walk							
Afternoon sunshine, 10-20+ min., depending on the season							
Pre-dinner berberine and ubiquinol							
Dinner at ____PM, incl. 2 cups plants							
Dinner salad							
Dinner finishes at ____PM							
Post-dinner 10 min. walk							
Switch to evening, dim-light mode at ____PM							
Take melatonin, 1 mg, about 2 hours before bed							
Supplements							
Take melatonin, 2 mg, right at bedtime							
In bed at ____PM							
Ovulation monitoring							
Sunday prep for next week							

Sunday planner

- ☐ Take your weekly measurements. See page 325 in the workbook.

- ☐ Read over Week 12's information.

- ☐ Put your five fasting days on your calendar.

- ☐ Review the information in your ProLon box.

- ☐ Plan Week 12's meals on page 258. (See page 331 for ideas.)

- ☐ Build Week 12's grocery list on page 259.

- ☐ Go grocery shopping (You can either go shopping on Sunday and buy items that will last until you finish your fast or postpone grocery shopping by a few days so your food doesn't go bad).

CHAPTER 15

Month 3, Week 12: Fasting

*J*t's your last week of fasting and your final week of the 12-week Fertility Fast Track!

I want to take a moment to commend you on the work you've done so far. Every change you have made in your life has been an investment in yourself, your family as it is today, and your family as it will become.

If there are parts of the plan that still feel hard or that you haven't figured out yet, circle back to those pieces as you move through this week and into the next phase of your fertility story.

This week, while you fast, I will show you how to get the rest of the toxins out of your home.

Switch to green cleaning supplies

The chemicals in household cleaning products enter your body in a variety of ways. They can absorb through your skin into your bloodstream. They can form a residue on surfaces such as tables and shelves and transfer to your hands and then the food you eat. Additionally, all of these products release fumes and scent-free particles into the air you breathe that are absorbed through the sensitive tissue in your lungs.

Volatile organic compounds (VOCs) are microscopic particles that evaporate or sublimate from solid and liquid substances. These compounds escape from cleaning solutions and other household products, such as paints and glues, and pollute the air you breathe.

VOC-emitting products are most active when wet, but they continue emitting VOCs long after a product is dry. So, when you use toxic products in your home, you continue to breathe them for days, weeks, or even years.

Indoor air pollution has a profound effect on human health. Research studies consistently find that exposure to VOCs and fine airborne particles increases headaches, sinus problems, and respiratory diseases like asthma.[1]

When it comes to fertility, women with higher blood levels of common household pollutants are more likely to take 12 months or longer to get pregnant, are more likely to have unexplained infertility, and when they do get pregnant, they are more likely to miscarry. On top of that, when pregnant women use household cleaning products, the more they use, the more likely it is that their children will have respiratory problems. In utero exposure to cleaning products damages developing fetal lung tissue.[2,3]

To lower these risks, make sure that all of your cleaning supplies are fragrance free, low-VOC, and non-toxic.

Tips:

- Check the safety of all of your household cleaners on the Environmental Working Group's Healthy Cleaning Guide (www. ewg.org/guides/cleaners). If a product is dangerous, get it out of your house. Some products are so toxic that you can't throw them away. You need to take them to a hazardous waste facility. Make sure you dispose of your chemicals properly.

- Store paints and solvents in your garage, not in your home.

- When you clean your home, your goal is to remove dirt. You don't need to disinfect your house. Avoid antimicrobials, disinfectants, bleach, and other powerful cleaners. In fact, when people over-sterilize their homes, they increase their risk of developing allergies and autoimmune diseases.

- In virtually all cases, you don't need commercial cleaners. For most surfaces, use a simple vinegar solution. Mix one cup of vinegar with one cup of water. Spray, wipe, done. If you need to give something a good scrubbing, use soap and a scrubber sponge with a paste of baking soda and water.

- If you do use a toxic cleaner (please don't!), wear gloves and a properly-rated mask, and thoroughly ventilate your workspace.

- Laundry detergent residue clings to clothes and stays in contact with your skin all day long. Make sure your detergent is fragrance free and nontoxic. Use oxygen bleach instead of chlorine bleach. Avoid dryer sheets altogether. Check all laundry products on the EWG database (www.ewg.org/guides/cleaners).

- Paint isn't a cleaner, but if you are ever painting a room, choose a zero-VOC paint. And for furniture, choose natural wood over engineered wood because the glue in engineered wood off-gases toxic VOCs.

Vacuum weekly

Cleaning products are just one source of industrial chemicals in our homes. Products such as couches and mattresses shed tiny pieces of foam. Carpets and curtains release chemically treated fibers. Electronics release tiny particles of flame retardants. All of these teensy tiny contaminants congregate in dust.

In 2015, a team of researchers from universities and environmental groups across the country came together to study household dust. They found that a typical indoor dust sample contains 45 different toxic chemicals and endocrine disruptors, including phthalates, flame retardants, and pesticides.[4,5]

These are the same chemicals that, when in food and personal care products, cause health ailments and female fertility problems.

Dust enters our bodies when we inhale it or when we touch it and then ingest it. Children and pets are most at risk because they spend so much time on the floor, and for children in particular, they put hands, toys, and pretty much everything in their mouths.

Get toxic dust out of your house! The best way to do this is to vacuum weekly with a high-efficiency particulate air (HEPA) filter vacuum cleaner.

Tips:

- Make sure your vacuum cleaner has a bag and a HEPA filter. Some of these hazardous particles are minute and you need to trap them in a filter. The worst vacuums are bagless because, instead of capturing these tiny contaminants, they circulate them into the air, and when you empty the vacuum canister, you get a plume of dust in your face. If your vacuum cleaner doesn't have a bag and a HEPA filter, you should replace it with one that does.

- After vacuuming, wipe all surfaces with a damp rag.

- If you are ever replacing the flooring in your home, choose natural hard surfaces such as wood, stone, or tile. Carpet collects dust and is often treated with toxic stain guards. Engineered wood and linoleum off-gas VOCs.

Clean your indoor air

You should do everything you can to limit the chemicals that come into your home, but you simply can't control everything.

Indoor air pollution is a part of modern life. In most locations, indoor pollution is worse than the air quality outside. The U.S. Environmental Protection Agency (EPA) estimates that most indoor air is two to five times more polluted than the air right outside the building. This is even more concerning when you consider than many people spend up to 90% of their time indoors.[6]

Poor indoor air quality raises your risk of cardiovascular disease, diabetes, and cancer, and it causes breathing problems and infections.

A HEPA air filter is your best tool for counteracting that risk. For adults and children with asthma and environmental allergies, HEPA filters reduce respiratory symptoms. Studies show that women who live in low-air-pollution environments are less likely to suffer from infertility than women who are exposed to high air pollution. Among pregnant women, exposure to air pollution increases rates of restricted fetal growth. Women in polluted cities who use indoor air filters give birth to healthier weight babies.[7,8]

A HEPA filter can remove 50% to 80% of airborne particles in a room and this can reduce your exposure to a wide range of chemicals. A whole home HEPA filter attached to your central heating and cooling system is the most efficient way to do this, but portable HEPA filters work great, too. You just need to make sure you have one powerful enough to clean the space it's in.

Run it day and night, even when you are not around.

Here are a few more tips to keep your indoor air clean and breathable.

Tips:

- Consider getting an extra HEPA air filter for your workplace.

- Follow your air filter manufacturer's guide and replace the HEPA filter on the recommended schedule.

- Any time you cook on your stove top, run the vent in the range hood. Gas stoves release nitrogen dioxide, which is a respiratory irritant. All cooking, and especially cooking at high heat, releases fine particles into the air that can damage lungs. Using the vent can reduce exposure by up to 90%.

- Test your home for radon. Current estimates are that one in five American homes has elevated radon levels. After tobacco smoke, it is the second leading cause of lung cancer in the United States. Pregnant women exposed to radon are more likely to give birth to babies with certain birth defects. You can't see or smell radon so you need to test your home to find out if you have a radon problem. Learn more here: www.cdc.gov/features/protect-home-radon.[10]

- Take care of any mold problems in your home. Mold releases spores into the air that people breathe. Called mycotoxins, some of these spores can cause a range of health problems, including respiratory illnesses, asthma, allergies, headaches, and fatigue. In severe cases, mycotoxins can cause poisoning, immune deficiency, and cancer.

- In all but the world's most polluted cities, the air outside is cleaner than the air inside. Whenever the weather allows, open your windows. Open every window you can, and if there's no breeze, use a fan to create one. Fill your indoor space with outdoor air.

Practice safe gardening

The chemicals used on the plants and spaces outside your home migrate into your home. They cling to shoes and clothes. They move in the air.

In your yard or garden, use organic fertilizers and do everything you can to avoid pesticides. For pest problems, try natural solutions first. Ladybugs eat aphids. You can get poison-free yellow jacket traps. Snails hate crushed eggshell, and ants hate cinnamon.

If you do use poisons, research eco-friendly pest control methods to find the safest options. The same goes for weed control.

You may also want to reconsider your attitude toward weeds and bugs. A couple of dandelions never killed anyone, but commercial weed killers and pesticides cause cancer.[11]

Tips:

- Landscape with native plant varieties that require less intensive gardening. You'll use fewer chemicals and less water, and you will save time and money. You will also provide food and habitat for native birds and insects.

- Homeowner Association (HOA) rules can basically require chemical-intensive gardening. Many people have successfully petitioned their HOAs to modernize their rules to be more water and eco-friendly.

- If you are a tenant, your rights regarding pesticide and herbicide sprays in the areas around your home vary place by place. Learn your rights. Most communities have resources for tenants as part of Housing and Urban Development (HUD).

- No matter how you garden, never wear outside shoes into your house. Pesticides, herbicides, and dust from roads can get tracked into your home on shoes. Take your shoes off at your front door, and if it's chilly, switch to indoor slippers.[12]

Week 12 organizer

Our homes shouldn't make us sick. We can't control everything, but we should make thoughtful choices about the products we buy and how we use them. Without going crazy or broke, do what you can to keep toxic chemicals out of your home and out of your body.

To-do list

☐ Check the safety of all of your home cleaning products by searching for them in the Environmental Working Group's Healthy Cleaning Guide (www.ewg.org/guides/cleaners).

☐ Purchase non-toxic cleaning supplies (vinegar, baking soda, a spray bottle, and a scrub pad).

☐ Buy a HEPA vacuum cleaner.

☐ Vacuum your whole house and wipe down surfaces with a damp cloth.

☐ Put HEPA air filters in the main living spaces in your home and consider getting another one for your workplace.

☐ Write to your HOA or landlord about pesticide and herbicide use.

☐   Test your home for radon.

☐   Take care of mold problems.

☐   Switch to organic gardening.

☐   Schedule and attend a yoga class, only if you feel up to it.

☐   Schedule and receive acupuncture or a massage.

Meal planner

* Don't forget to plan a fancy Sunday brunch to celebrate the end of your fast.

	Breakfast	Lunch	Dinner	Misc
Mon	ProLon	ProLon	ProLon	ProLon
Tues	ProLon	ProLon	ProLon	ProLon
Wed	ProLon	ProLon	ProLon	ProLon
Thurs	ProLon	ProLon	ProLon	ProLon
Fri	ProLon	ProLon	ProLon	ProLon
Sat				
Sun				

Grocery list

* Because you are fasting this week, you only need food for your two non-fasting days. If you are not fasting, use the same shopping list from last week.

☐ Greens, enough for two days

☐ Salad stuff, enough for two days

☐ ½ pound of dried beans, any type

☐ Soup, broth or tomato based, not cream based (choose boxes or jars instead of cans, or plan to make your own from scratch), for your first post-fast meals

☐ Spearmint tea

_____

_____

_____

_____

_____

_____

_____

_____

_____

_____

_____

_____

_____

Daily checklist

* Here is your final fasting–week checklist.

	M	T	W	Th	F	Sa	Su
Wake up at ____AM							
ProLon breakfast at ____ AM							
Post-breakfast 10 minute walk							
Morning sunshine, 20-30 minutes							
ProLon lunch							
Post-lunch 10 minute walk							
ProLon dinner finishes at ____PM							
Post-dinner 10 minute walk							
Switch to evening, dim-light mode at ____PM							
Take melatonin, 1 mg, about 2 hours before bed							
Take melatonin, 2 mg, right at bedtime							
In bed at ____PM							
Ovulation monitoring							

You're done! Well...sort of.

There is no Sunday Planner at the end of this week because, at the end of Week 12, you are officially finished with the 12-Week Fertility Fast Track program. This is an unbelievably wonderful achievement!

You are done...but not really done. In fact, this is really just a beginning. It's now time to plan the next steps in your fertility journey. And to move forward, you have to keep all of the health that you've gained.

Even though you are finished with the Fertility Fast Track program, you should continue to follow the protocol. If you go back to your previous way of living, your body will return to its previous state of health.

On Sunday of Week 12, go on to the next chapter in this book, "What happens next;" at the end, on page 283, there is a template weekly organizer that you can use to plan out future weeks.

CHAPTER 16

What happens next

*Y*ou have made it through the 12-week Fertility Fast Track program! This is a monumental accomplishment. The investment that you have made in yourself and your health is invaluable.

Whether you have followed this program perfectly or imperfectly, please take a moment to acknowledge and honor what you have done. Before you move forward, stop and fully appreciate your body as it is today.

No matter what happens next, this is your body. You cannot exist without it. Whether or not you get pregnant in the upcoming weeks or months, please give your body the love, gratitude, and forgiveness it has always deserved.

How pregnancy happens

As you make plans for the future, you should maintain your new healthy habits. All of your Fertility Fast Track schedules—your eating schedule, fasting schedule, sleeping schedule, light-dark schedule, and exercise schedule—are still relevant and important. Your highly nutritious, high-fiber diet is more essential than ever. Continue to diligently avoid endocrine disruptors and environmental toxins. The same strategies that helped you improve your health will help you get pregnant, have a safe pregnancy and delivery, and set the foundation for a lifetime of wellness for your baby.

In order to get pregnant the old-fashioned way, a sequence of highly coordinated events must occur in your body.

1. **Ovulation:** A healthy egg is recruited in one of your ovaries to fully mature. The quality of your egg depends heavily on proper nutrition and minimal to no inflammation or oxidative stress in the ovary. When the egg is ready, a spike in estrogen causes a peak in LH, which triggers the egg to burst from its follicle. This is ovulation.

2. **Fertilization:** The egg enters the fallopian tube. It takes about 12 to 24 hours for the egg to travel down the fallopian tube toward the uterus. During this time, if the egg encounters a sperm, the sperm enters the egg and fertilization occurs. Your egg must be fertilized when it is in your fallopian tube, not in your uterus. This is why your peak fertility occurs in the two to three days before ovulation; after ovulation you only have those 12 to 24 hours to get pregnant before the egg leaves the fallopian tube. Sperm can live up to six days so give them a head start. Have unprotected sex every other day during the week before ovulation so sperm are ready and waiting in your fallopian tubes when your egg arrives. If the egg travels all the way down the fallopian tube into the uterus without encountering sperm, it will disintegrate and you will menstruate two weeks later.

3. **Cell division:** At the moment of fertilization, the egg becomes a zygote. No more sperm can enter. The zygote hangs out in the fallopian tube for three to four days and begins a period of rapid cell division.

4. **Implantation:** When the zygote finally reaches the uterus, the uterine wall should be nice and thick. The zygote will burrow into the uterine wall. This is when pregnancy begins. The zygote becomes a blastocyst and forms the placenta, which releases progesterone and prevents menstruation.

5. **Pregnancy:** In addition to progesterone, the placenta produces human chorionic gonadotropin (hCG). This is the hormone that a home pregnancy test screens for. About seven days after implantation (almost two weeks after ovulation), hCG can be detected in urine. This is the earliest point at which you can get a positive pregnancy test.

6. **Ultrasound Pregnancy:** At around five or six weeks, your doctor will be able to confirm your pregnancy on an ultrasound. This is a significant milestone. As many as 25% of all pregnancies end before five weeks due to abnormalities in the blastocyst or the woman's body. Early miscarriages are called chemical pregnancies because they produce positive pregnancy tests but never progress to a physically detectable pregnancy. Once a doctor can see your pregnancy on an ultrasound, your risk of miscarriage begins a steady week-by-week decline.[1]

For women with PCOS, every step of this pregnancy process is more likely to go wrong. Lack of ovulation is the biggest impediment to pregnancy, but that's not the sole challenge. PCOS women tend to have lower quality eggs, which lowers fertilization and implantation success rates and increases miscarriage rates. On top of that, our hormone levels and rhythms are not quite the same as those of non-PCOS women, which further contributes to our much higher rates of miscarriage.

For most PCOS women, it makes sense to try to get pregnant by living the healthiest lifestyle you can and having frequent unprotected sex timed to your fertility window. However, there are a variety of reasons why some couples, even if they do everything "right," will need fertility treatments to achieve pregnancy and a baby.

Different fertility treatments step in and bolster different stages of the pregnancy process. Some induce ovulation. Some handle the entire process up to implantation. Only a doctor working intimately with a woman and her partner can decide which assisted reproductive technology (ART) treatment is most appropriate.

Every step of the Fertility Fast Track program is designed to improve your chances of success at all stages of the pregnancy process, no matter how you try to conceive. What you do next depends on exactly how your body responded over these past 12 weeks plus other factors such as your age, medical history, and the medical history of your partner.

Your next steps

I can provide some guidelines on how to approach trying to conceive, but if you are unclear about what makes the most sense in your unique situation, you should make a follow-up appointment with your doctor.

Spend a few more months on the Fertility Fast Track program.

Where is your health today? If you are making progress on the Fertility Fast Track, but your health metrics aren't where you want them yet, consider giving your body another month or more of preconception care. I especially recommend this for women who are seeing health improvements, but still have worrisome health metrics:

- BMI above 25
- High blood pressure
- High fasting glucose

These risk factors will make it harder to get pregnant and they will make pregnancy more dangerous for you and your baby. Consider giving your body a few more months of healing.

This is also an appropriate strategy for women who are seeing health improvements but have not yet started ovulating regularly.

At the end of this chapter, I have included a Weekly Organizer that captures the culmination of the 12-week program. You can use this organizer for as long as you stay on the program. Follow the program schedule for three weeks; then do another round of the Fasting Mimicking Diet on the fourth week. You can continue this plan—three weeks of the Fertility Fast Track and one week of the Fasting Mimicking Diet, repeating—for up to a year, and then you should switch to the long-term maintenance supplement program (page 287), just so you don't stay on high-dose supplements forever. As long as you are doing the Fasting Mimicking Diets, you should avoid pregnancy. Extended fasting and pregnancy are not a safe combination.

Of course, your decision to invest more time in preconception care needs to be balanced with the inherent risks of delaying pregnancy and getting older.

If you are older than 35, you need to weigh the benefits of increased health and fertility with the natural decrease in fertility that occurs over time. In general, for most people, the benefits of improved health and fertility more than make up for the loss of fertility that happens over another few months.

In most cases, repeating the program for three more months is a sensible compromise. But every situation is unique. You should discuss with your doctor what makes the most sense for you and your family.

Try to get pregnant naturally.
If you are ovulating and in good health, if your partner has normal fertility, and if your doctor hasn't identified any reasons you shouldn't attempt pregnancy, then you should try to conceive naturally. Natural

pregnancies are the safest, lowest risk pregnancies for mothers and babies. For most couples, this is where you should start.

Stay on the Fertility Fast Track diet and lifestyle program, using the Weekly Organizer at the end of this chapter. Continue fasting overnight for 13 hours, sleeping seven to eight hours every night, eating well, exercising regularly, and taking all of your supplements. In addition to improving your overall health, many of these supplements and lifestyle routines specifically improve your chances of successful fertilization and implantation. Just don't do any more Fasting Mimicking Diets because extended fasting and pregnancy don't mix.

Monitor your menstrual cycle and keep an eye on physical fertility signs. Remember that your cervical mucus will be clear and stretchy like egg whites on your most fertile days. Then have unprotected sex every other day throughout your fertile window—the five days before ovulation and the day of ovulation.

When you have trying-to-conceive sex, so long as your partner ejaculates into your vagina, you are doing it right. Here's what the research says about baby-making:

- No position is better than any other. Healthy sperm are great swimmers. It takes about 15 minutes for them to travel from your vagina to your fallopian tubes. In studies, sexual position does not seem to affect this. If you want to lie on your back and put a pillow under your hips so that gravity gives the little guys an extra nudge, you certainly won't hurt anything, but it's not necessary.[2]

- You don't need to orgasm to get pregnant. Female orgasm seems to help sperm along their journey, but they can get to your fallopian tubes just fine without one. There are no statistical differences in pregnancy rates between women who do and don't orgasm. If you orgasm, great, and if not, don't worry about it.[3]

- If you are one of the approximately 40% of women who use a vaginal lubricant during sex, make sure you choose a sperm-friendly brand such as Pre-Seed. Most commercially available lubricants reduce sperm mobility by between 60% and 100%, making it much harder for them to reach your fallopian tubes.

Beyond that, it takes time and luck. A couple with average fertility has about a 20% chance of getting pregnant each ovulation cycle. That means that more than half of couples with no fertility challenges will get pregnant within three cycles. But many will take longer; it's just human biology.

How long should *you* try to conceive before moving on to the world of fertility treatments? A general rule of thumb is one year for women younger than 35 and six months for women 35 or older.

Conduct additional testing.

When I have a patient who has what is typically classified as "unexplained infertility," I always run a few more tests before I refer her to a fertility treatment center. Unexplained fertility doesn't mean that there isn't a cause; it simply means we doctors haven't figured it out. There are many additional tests that can be ordered by your primary care physician or a doctor at a fertility clinic. Some tests that have changed the course of my patients' treatments are:

- **Autoimmunity and allergy testing:** Autoimmune disease often plays a role in female infertility. Cyrex Laboratories (www. cyrexlabs.com/CyrexTestsArrays) offers a wide range of tests that can help pinpoint autoimmune diseases, allergies, and sensitivities. Array 11, Chemical Immune Reactivity Screen, and Array 12, Pathogen-Associated Immune Reactivity Screen, often reveal surprising immune responses to environmental toxins and chemicals.

- **Celiac testing:** A standard celiac panel can produce a false negative. For patients with persistent infertility, I often order more sensitive celiac testing from Vibrant America because they test for advanced markers of gluten autoimmunity and leaky gut (www.vibrant-america.com/celiac-disease).

- **Environmental toxic chemical exposures testing:** High blood levels of any number of toxic chemicals and endocrine disruptors can impact female fertility. I use Genova Diagnostics to test my patients for exposure to toxic chemicals such as BPA, phthalates, and solvents and to heavy metals. You can order the tests individually, but I usually order these three panels, which cover a wide range of toxins that have known detrimental effects on female health and fertility:
    - Bisphenol A (BPA) Profile (www.gdx.net/product/bisphenol-a-bpa-test-urine)
    - Toxic Effects CORE panel (www.gdx.net/product/toxic-effects-core-test-urine-blood)
    - Toxic Metals - Whole Blood panel (www.gdx.net/product/toxic-metals-test-blood)

- **Fertility Profile and Menstrual Mapping:** To better understand and track a patient's hormones throughout her menstrual cycle, I will order panels from ZRT Laboratory (www.zrtlab.com/test-specialties). For PCOS patients, the Fertility Panel and Menstrual Mapping are most useful. The most common condition I find is progesterone deficiency during the luteal phase of the menstrual cycle, which makes it harder to get pregnant. This can be corrected with progesterone supplementation.

- **Inflammation markers testing:** Inflammation is a foundational component of PCOS and impacts your fertility in a variety of invisible ways. I order the Inflammation Panel through Cleveland Heart Lab (www.clevelandheartlab.com/test-menu).

- **Reproductive Cavity Screening:** There are several different types of imaging tests that can screen for anatomical abnormalities in your uterus and other reproductive organs. Your doctor will advise you on the best test for you and your situation. This will be an in-person exam, and your doctor will tell you where to go to have it performed.

- **Semen analysis:** If your partner has already had a semen analysis performed, he may also want to request the SpermComet test (examenlab.com/healthcare-professionals/about-spermcomet-test), which analyzes a semen sample for high rates of DNA damage. This is a much more sensitive test than the standard male fertility test, and if it comes back abnormal, you will need to work closely with a fertility clinic to devise the best strategies for achieving pregnancy. (And if your partner didn't follow the protocol in this book, he should. Male health is an essential part of the pregnancy equation. My friend, colleague, and esteemed fertility expert, Professor Tremellen wrote a bonus section on male fertility that your partner should read, beginning on page 293, if he hasn't already.)

Begin fertility treatments.

If you are not menstruating, if you are menstruating but you can't get pregnant, or if you've had more than one miscarriage, it may be time to contact a fertility center.

Make sure that you choose a clinic that understands the unique needs of PCOS women. I cannot emphasize this enough. We respond differently to many common treatments. If you want the best shot of getting pregnant with the smallest risk of painful, scary side effects, you need a doctor who understands the unique physiology of PCOS women.

Some of the topics you should discuss with your fertility doctor:

- **Ovarian hyperstimulation syndrome (OHSS):** OHSS is a potential side effect of any ovary-stimulating procedure, including ovulation induction, intrauterine insemination, and IVF. When a woman's ovaries become hyperstimulated, they become swollen and painful. Most cases are minor, but in severe situations, this condition can lead to kidney failure and death. Polycystic ovaries increase the risk for OHSS, and consequently, PCOS women have double the rate of OHSS. Find out how your doctor plans to lower your OHSS risk and monitor you.[4]

- **Letrozole (LEH-troh-zole) vs. Clomid:** Both of these pharmaceuticals can induce ovulation, but in general, women with

PCOS respond better to letrozole than Clomid. Although Clomid is the standard first-line treatment for anovulation, as many as 40% of PCOS women are Clomid-resistant. Women with PCOS who take letrozole have a 55% higher birth rate than PCOS women who take Clomid. In some cases, PCOS women who are resistant to both letrozole and Clomid will successfully ovulate when both drugs are combined. If you are going to attempt ovulation induction, discuss drug options with your doctor.[5,6,7,8]

- **Metformin vs. myo-inositol:** Metformin is a pharmaceutical competitor to myo-inositol that sensitizes your body to insulin. For lean PCOS women, metformin outperforms Clomid for helping PCOS women get pregnant. However, I do not recommend metformin as a fertility treatment. Metformin is a powerful endocrine disruptor, and children exposed to metformin in-utero have increased rates of metabolic disease. In a study published in 2018, children born to PCOS mothers who took metformin during pregnancy had almost double the rate of childhood obesity compared to children whose PCOS mothers did not take metformin. By age four, 32% of the metformin children were overweight or obese. Metformin simply isn't safe for pregnancy, but this information is so new that your doctor may not know it. I strongly prefer myo-inositol over metformin. In studies, PCOS women are equally successful in achieving pregnancy on myo-inositol as they are on metformin, but myo-inositol is not an endocrine disruptor. If you and your doctor decide that metformin is the best option for you, discuss a plan to stop taking metformin as soon as you get pregnant.[9,10]

- **Liraglutide:** Liraglutide is a glucagon-like peptide-1 receptor agonist sold under the brand names Victoza and Saxenda. It is an injectable drug that induces rapid, significant weight-loss. Overweight and obese PCOS women who take liraglutide for six to seven months will lose, on average, 20 pounds. Consequently, many fertility centers recommend that overweight and obese PCOS women take liraglutide for several months before starting fertility treatments. This increases your chances of becoming pregnant, having a healthy pregnancy, and delivering a healthy baby. I think this is a reasonable treatment, but obviously, it is a quick-fix that doesn't permanently fix anything. To keep the weight off, you still need to adopt a healthy lifestyle like the one described in this book.[11]

- **Gonadotropins, IUI, and IVF:** If you move on to more invasive procedures, such as injectable gonadotropins, intrauterine insemination (IUI), and in vitro fertilization (IVF), make sure you understand the costs and the risks. Ask about the success rates specifically for PCOS women because, in general, they are lower than for non-PCOS women.

No matter what fertility treatments you pursue, stay on the Fertility Fast Track schedule, diet, and supplements program. These interventions increase your chances of getting pregnant through assisted reproductive technology. Do everything except the Fasting Mimicking Diet; no extended fasting while you try to get pregnant.

Negative pregnancy tests

Every attempt at pregnancy is a tiny, fragile hope, and every negative pregnancy test shatters that hope anew. Most couples experience several negative pregnancy tests as they build their families. Some couples experience a lot. There's no fairness. It just is what it is.

And for many people, it hurts.

Take care of yourself through this period. Love yourself. Love your partner. Invest in your relationships. Don't put your life on hold.

If your emotional state feels unhealthy, seek out help and support.

- Invest in self-care, such as massage, acupuncture, and daily guided imagery.
- Find a therapist who can help you understand and process your emotions.

- Join an online community. My favorites are Path2Parenthood (www.path2parenthood.org) and Resolve (resolve.org).
- Frequently reconnect with your partner and your loved ones.
- Have fun, make plans, and start new things.

As you try to build your family, don't lose yourself.

Pregnancy

When you get that positive pregnancy test, it can feel like sunshine, singing, and cotton candy. There really aren't words to describe the joy, disbelief, and fear that simultaneously explode from your heart when you hold a positive pregnancy test in your shaking hand.

Savor it in all of its complexity.

And then move into pregnancy mode. Pregnancy mode looks a lot like the Fertility Fast Track program, but with a few key differences.

First and foremost, no extended fasting. Definitely no more Fasting Mimicking Diets. But continue your overnight fasts. I recommend 12 hours because in studies, pregnant women who fast for 12 hours every night have a lower risk of developing gestational diabetes.[12]

Adjust your supplements protocol. As soon as you get your positive pregnancy test, stop taking berberine and curcumin. If you are taking resveratrol, ubiquinol, or any hemp or cannabis products, including CBD, stop taking those as well.

If you are not taking one of the prenatal vitamins I recommend—Pure Encapsulations PreNatal Nutrients or Thorne Basic Prenatal—look over the ingredients and make sure your prenatal has folate (not folic acid), iodine, iron, vitamin E, and zinc.

Talk to your doctor about the supplements you may want to take during your pregnancy. In addition to your prenatal vitamin, you may want to consider taking these supplements from the Fertility Fast Track program:

- **Myo-inositol:** 4 g / 4000 mg in a glass of water
- **NAC:** 600 mg to 1800 mg
- **Omega-3:** 1 dose, with at least 600 mg EPA and 400 mg DHA
- **Probiotic:** 1 dose
- **Quercetin:** 250 mg
- **Vaginal probiotic:** 1 dose
- **Vitamin D3:** 2000 mg (adjust down if your prenatal already includes vitamin D)

You should also consider adding a few new supplements:

- **Choline:** Most prenatal vitamins, including the ones I recommend, do not include this nutrient that is essential for proper fetal brain development. I recommend that pregnant women take 950 mg per day. In a study from 2017, when pregnant women took just over 900 mg per day of choline, their babies were smarter and could think faster than women who took the standard recommended dose of 480 mg per day. I give my patients Thorne Phosphatidyl Choline (2 capsules daily) or Douglas Laboratories Choline Bitartrate (4 capsules daily).[13]

- **Magnesium:** You should aim to get about 400 mg of magnesium every day. Magnesium lowers rates of preeclampsia and other pregnancy complications. See what your prenatal has and supplement appropriately. The two prenatals I recommend have under 100 mg. I give my patients Pure Encapsulations Magnesium Glycinate or UltraMag Magnesium. The UltraMag Magnesium has higher bioavailability so you only need to take one capsule.[14]

Studies seem to indicate that these supplements at these dosages are safe and beneficial during pregnancy. As with all medicinally active compounds, sometimes researchers discover negative side effects years down the line.

I highly recommend that you discuss your personal risk factors with your doctor and decide which supplements will likely benefit you the most.

Because PCOS women have higher rates of pregnancy complications, you should also discuss what health metrics you should monitor and what symptoms warrant a call to your doctor's office. I suggest that all pregnant PCOS women monitor:

- **Blood pressure:** Take your blood pressure daily. You are watching for early signs of hypertension that could lead to preeclampsia, a dangerous pregnancy complication marked by extremely high blood pressure. Take this measurement around 8PM after sitting and resting for 10 minutes. If you notice a significant increase from your pre-pregnancy blood pressure (+30 on the top number or +15 on the bottom number) or if your blood pressure ever exceeds 140/90, you should contact your doctor.

- **Blood sugar:** Unless you have diabetes, it's hard to monitor this on your own. Because you are at higher risk of gestational diabetes, you should ask your doctor to test you for elevated blood sugar earlier than normal. Most women get their glucose tolerance tested between 24 and 28 weeks. All PCOS women should have an additional earlier test done at around 12 to 14 weeks. If you already have diabetes or are at exceptionally high risk of gestational diabetes, consider getting a continuous glucose monitor (CGM). In studies, diabetic pregnant women who use CGMs have better blood sugar control and better pregnancy outcomes compared to women who do traditional capillary glucose monitoring.[15]

At any point, if you have pain or bleeding, contact your doctor. In the third trimester when most pregnancy complications develop, let your doctor know right away if you notice:

- Abdominal pain, particularly in the upper right quadrant
- Contractions, more frequently than 10 minutes apart
- Decreased baby movement or kick count
- Fluid, leaking or gushing
- Headaches, abnormally sudden or severe

- Swelling, anywhere and particularly in the hands and feet
- Weight gain, abnormally rapid

Or anything that doesn't feel "right." Trust in the wisdom of your body to know if something is wrong and don't worry about bothering your doctor. Your doctor is there to help you have a healthy pregnancy. Answering questions is part of our job. Any abnormal symptom could be a sign of a health condition. Your doctor will let you know if she thinks she should examine and monitor you.

If your doctor ever says you are fine or your symptoms are normal but you still feel like something is wrong, go get a second opinion. Doctors make mistakes. No doctor should ever be insulted by a patient who gets a second opinion. Throughout your pregnancy, delivery, and beyond, be your own best health advocate.

Miscarriage

Pregnancy loss or miscarriage is a normal part of human reproduction. It is the female body's way of ending a pregnancy that isn't viable.

All women are at risk of miscarriage, but women with PCOS are at higher risk than non-PCOS women, and we are more likely to experience recurrent pregnancy loss. This is due to a variety of factors:[16]

- Lower egg quality means that there are more likely to be abnormalities in the embryo.
- Concurrent medical conditions such as obesity, diabetes, and vascular disease can disrupt pregnancy progression.[17]
- Any hormonal imbalance, including hyperandrogenism, can contribute to pregnancy loss.[18]
- High blood levels of endocrine disrupting chemicals are linked to higher rates of miscarriage.[19]

If you notice pain or bleeding, notify your doctor right away, but recognize that once a miscarriage begins, there is nothing anyone can do to stop it. In most cases, the miscarriage was inevitable from the beginning. Pregnancy is complicated and there are many opportunities for things to go wrong.

At the end of the day, one miscarriage, as heartrending as it is, is considered normal.

If you have a miscarriage, your doctor will guide you through the process. Depending on how far along you are, you may or may not need medical intervention. The most common ways of treating miscarriage are:

- **Expectant management:** This is essentially wait and see. If a pregnancy ends before 10 weeks, most women's bodies will naturally expel all of the uterine pregnancy tissue. The miscarriage will feel like a heavy period. The farther along a woman is, the more tissue she will pass. The heaviest bleeding lasts about three to five hours and lighter bleeding can last up to two weeks.

- **Medical management:** A doctor may prescribe misoprostol (Cytotec) when a woman has lost a pregnancy, as indicated by lack of a fetal heartbeat, but has not begun to pass the pregnancy tissue. This pharmaceutical triggers the uterine lining to shed. Misoprostol can also help in cases where a miscarriage is incomplete and an ultrasound shows tissue remaining in a woman's uterus.

- **Dilation and curettage (D&C):** A D&C is a common and minor surgical procedure where a doctor dilates a woman's cervix and uses an instrument to remove tissue from her uterus. A D&C is usually recommended for later miscarriages because they are less likely to complete on their own. After a D&C, a woman can experience bleeding for up to two weeks, but usually less, and there shouldn't be any large clots.

A woman should discuss these options with her doctor and make the best choice for her physical and emotional health. Some of my patients want to experience their miscarriage naturally and some need to move through the miscarriage before they can begin healing. This is a personal decision.

After a miscarriage, take care of your body, your mind, and your heart. When you lose a pregnancy, all of them hurt.

- Watch for complications. Call your doctor or go to the emergency room if you experience bleeding that lasts longer than two weeks, heavy bleeding, pain beyond normal menstrual cramping, abnormal discharge, or fever. This could be a sign of an infection or an incomplete miscarriage.

- Wait two weeks and until the bleeding has stopped before having sex or putting anything in your vagina.

- Wait at least one menstrual cycle before you try to get pregnant again. There's a slightly elevated risk of miscarriage in pregnancies that occur in the first menstrual cycle following a miscarriage.

- Throughout this process and for as long as you need to, take special care of your emotional health and reestablish your mind-body connection. Get massages. Practice guided imagery. As soon as you feel able, return to yoga classes.

- Find a therapist who specializes in pregnancy loss.

- Many communities have in-person pregnancy loss support groups that can provide a safe space for you to discuss your feelings and experiences.

- Explore online resources. Share—Pregnancy and Infant Loss Support (nationalshare.org) is an excellent place to start.

Recurrent miscarriage

One miscarriage is considered normal but two or more may indicate a medical problem. If you have two or more miscarriages, I recommend that you work with a fertility specialist to investigate the cause.

Earlier in this chapter, I listed out additional tests (page 269) that can shed light on persistent fertility issues. You should get all of these tests done. You may also want to consider:

- **Genetic screening:** In up to 5% of couples experiencing recurrent miscarriage, one or both of the parents have a genetic anomaly called a chromosomal translocation. In many cases, the only symptom is recurrent pregnancy loss. This can be diagnosed with a genetic test called a karyotype (KARE-ee-oh-type). Most couples with a chromosomal translocation will eventually have a successful pregnancy, but they may experience several miscarriages first. Some couples may choose to use IVF so they can screen fertilized eggs for the chromosomal abnormality and only implant healthy zygotes.

- **Genetic testing of miscarriage tissue:** Discuss with your doctor whether you might gain additional useful information by performing a genetic test on your miscarriage tissue. In some cases of recurrent pregnancy loss, both parents will have normal genetic karyotype results, but they will still produce a high number of embryos with karyotype errors. The only way to know if this is happening is to test the embryo itself. Couples who produce a high percentage of abnormal embryos may benefit from IVF where the fertilized eggs can be tested for genetic anomalies before implantation. Conversely, in cases of repeat miscarriages where no genetic anomalies are detected, this could signal a harder to detect parental condition. For example, some women experience recurrent pregnancy loss because of anticoagulant and antiphospholipid antibody disorders. For this test, I recommend Natera because they provide results that are not impacted by maternal cell contamination (www.natera.com/anora-miscarriage-test). You will need to ask your doctor to order the test kit. If you collect the pregnancy tissue at home you will need a sterile container to collect and store it in. Consequently, it is a good idea to discuss miscarriage genetic testing with your doctor before you have a miscarriage.

- **Progesterone supplementation:** In women with multiple miscarriages, progesterone supplementation through the first 12 weeks of pregnancy may reduce the risk of subsequent miscarriages.[20]

Most couples who experience recurrent pregnancy losses will eventually have a successful pregnancy and live birth, but while you are going through it, repeated miscarriages are immensely painful and frustrating.

There's nothing I can say that will make this process feel okay. Give yourself permission to grieve every loss. Take time for you and your family to heal. Make decisions that best honor your heart, mind, and body.

Rates of depression among women experiencing multiple miscarriages are three times as high as they are in women without a history of miscarriage. Work with a trusted therapist and continue to live the healthiest lifestyle you can. Not only will following the Fertility Fast Track program give you your best shot for a successful pregnancy, it will support your mental health as well.[21]

And through it all, stay engaged in the rest of your life. Decide what that means to you, and then do it. Don't stop living.

Prioritize healthy living

No matter what your next steps are, the Fertility Fast Track program will make you healthier and increase your chances for success. Continue to follow the protocol to the best of your ability.

Female fertility is a sign of overall female health. At its core, this Fertility Fast Track program is designed to help you attain optimal health. This is excellent for your fertility, and equally importantly, it is fabulous for you.

Because you are more than your ovaries and uterus. You are a whole, vibrant, powerful woman.

Stay on the Fertility Fast Track program. Do it for your future family, no matter what it looks like. And do it for yourself.

Sometimes it takes a goal like getting pregnant to trigger a change in our lives. Embrace your hope for a pregnancy and a baby, but at the same time, invest in your health for you. Whether you get pregnant or not, you are enough as you are.

You are worth the time, expense, and effort.

Be healthy for you.

Weekly organizer

Now that you've completed the 12-week Fertility Fast Track program, use this organizer to maintain your healthy new habits and plan out upcoming weeks.

To-do list

☐ Vacuum your whole house and wipe down surfaces with a damp cloth.

☐ Schedule and attend one to three yoga classes.

☐ Schedule and receive acupuncture or a massage.

Meal planner

* Avoid added sugar, gluten, highly processed foods, and alcohol.
* Limit caffeine to one eight ounce beverage and limit meat to one small serving per day.
* Drink 70 mL (about one-third of a cup) of beetroot juice with breakfast daily.
* Eat a quarter-cup of fermented foods once a day.
* Drink two cups of spearmint tea every day.
* Include a serving of soy three to four times per week.

	Breakfast	Lunch	Dinner	Misc
Mon				
Tues				
Wed				
Thurs				
Fri				
Sat				
Sun				

Grocery list

- ☐ Greens, 1 pound carton of prewashed mixed salad greens

- ☐ Salad accessories (veggies, fruits, nuts, dressing)

- ☐ 2 pounds of dried beans, any type

- ☐ Fruits to be eaten as side dishes (apples, pears, berries, grapes, melons)

- ☐ Cold veggie sides (carrot sticks, cherry tomatoes, olives)

- ☐ Warm veggie sides (potatoes, yams, squash, Brussels sprouts, asparagus, green beans)

- ☐ Dark chocolate (dark chocolate covered almonds, 90% cacao bar, dark chocolate chips)

- ☐ Beetroot juice

- ☐ Fermented foods (sauerkraut and kimchi; if you eat dairy, also plain whole milk yogurt and kefir)

- ☐ Soy (tofu, tempeh, edamame)

- ☐ Spearmint tea

_____

_____

_____

_____

_____

_____

_____

Daily checklist

	M	T	W	Th	F	Sa	Su
Eat 1 cup of beans, anytime							
Eat ¼ cup of fermented veggies, anytime							
Drink 2 cups of spearmint tea, anytime							
15-30 minutes of guided imagery, anytime							
Wake up at ____AM							
Pre-breakfast berberine, ubiquinol, and nitric oxide							
Breakfast at ____AM, incl. 2 cups plants and 70 mL beetroot juice							
Post-breakfast 10 minute walk							
Morning sunshine, 20-30 minutes							
Pre-lunch berberine, ubiquinol, and nitric oxide							
Lunch, incl. 2 cups plants							
Post-lunch 10 minute walk							
Afternoon sunshine, 10-20+ minutes, depending on the season							
Pre-dinner berberine and ubiquinol							
Dinner at ____PM, incl. 2 cups plants							
Dinner salad							
Dinner finishes at ____PM							
Post-dinner 10 minute walk							
Switch to evening, dim-light mode at ____PM							
Take melatonin, 1 mg, about 2 hours before bed							
Supplements							
Take melatonin, 2 mg, right at bedtime							
In bed at ____PM							
Ovulation monitoring							

Daily supplements protocol

This is the complete supplement protocol, including the additional recommendations from Week 11 (page 240).

Before Breakfast
- Berberine: 500 mg
- Ubiquinol: 200 mg
- Nitric oxide: 1 dose

Before Lunch
- Berberine: 500 mg
- Ubiquinol: 200 mg
- Nitric oxide: 1 dose

Before Dinner
- Berberine: 500 mg
- Ubiquinol: 200 mg

Before Bed
- Mix 2 scoops of myo-inositol (4 g / 4000 mg) into a glass of water and take...
- Curcumin: 1500 mg
- NAC: 1800 mg
- Omega-3: 1 dose, with at least 600 mg EPA and 400 mg DHA
- Prenatal: 1 dose
- Probiotic: 1 dose
- Quercetin: 1000 mg
- Resveratrol: 40 mg
- Vaginal probiotic: 1 dose
- Vitamin D3: 2000 mg (adjust down if your prenatal already includes vitamin D)

Daily supplements protocol, after one year

* After one year, you should reduce the dosage on a few of the supplements
- Curcumin: Reduce from 1500 mg to 500 mg
- NAC: Reduce from 1800 mg to 900 mg
- Quercetin: Reduce from 1000 mg to 500 mg

Daily Supplements Protocol, after positive pregnancy test
* Consult with your doctor about what supplements to take during pregnancy in addition to your daily prenatal multivitamin. Supplements are medically active compounds. Studies seem to indicate that the supplements I recommend at the dosages provided are safe and beneficial during pregnancy. However, it is always possible that researchers will discover negative side effects in the future. I highly recommend that you discuss your personal risk factors with your doctor and decide which supplements will likely benefit you the most.

Definitely *stop* taking:
- Berberine
- Curcumin
- Resveratrol
- Ubiquinol
- Cannabis (any marijuana, hemp, or CBD product)

Consider taking these supplements from the Fertility Fast Track program:
- Myo-inositol: 4 g / 4000 mg in a glass of water and take...
- NAC: 600 mg to 1800 mg
- Omega-3: 1 dose, with at least 600 mg EPA and 400 mg DHA
- Probiotic: 1 dose
- Quercetin: 250 mg
- Vaginal probiotic: 1 dose
- Vitamin D3: 2000 mg (adjust down if your prenatal already includes vitamin D)

Consider adding these additional supplements:
- Choline: 480 mg to 950 mg
- Magnesium: 400 mg (adjust down if your prenatal already includes magnesium)

CHAPTER 17

Conclusion

*T*rying to start a family is an exciting, emotional time in life. For women struggling with PCOS and infertility, it can also be frustrating and heartbreaking.

PCOS is a complex disorder that is profoundly exacerbated by modern-day culture and diet. Fertility challenges are only one small piece of the modern PCOS condition.

To heal your fertility, you need to heal the entirety of your PCOS. It's hard work and it means being deeply thoughtful about your diet and lifestyle.

If you want to be healthy and fertile, you can't eat sugar and gluten. You can't spend your days indoors, stay out late, and drink alcohol. You can't live a modern western lifestyle and eat a modern western diet. It will make you sick. It will steal your fertility.

People did not evolve living this way. Modern culture is a relatively recent product of modern technology. No one really thrives when they live a modern life—working inside, spending a lot of time in front of screens, eating processed convenience foods, and going to bed well after sundown. It's true that some people do okay, but if you have PCOS, you are not one of those people.

I carefully designed the PCOS SOS Fertility Fast Track program specifically for my PCOS patients to recreate a healthy, natural lifestyle and diet that can coexist with the modern toxic world that we all must survive in.

When you heal from PCOS, when you turn a modern-day disease-like syndrome back into a historic, mild difference, you rediscover the incredible strength and vitality that your PCOS foremothers passed down to you.

PCOS women are strong. We are fighters and survivors. That is both our legacy and our destiny.

PCOS never goes away entirely. But when you get healthy, PCOS transforms from a disease into just one aspect of your unique and wonderful body.

I truly hope that sometime soon, in the next few weeks or months, you will become pregnant and give birth to a healthy baby.

There are no guarantees in life. Every woman and her partner are different, and every story of fertility and family-building is unique.

I have worked with thousands of women, and the vast majority of my patients who follow my health advice restore their fertility, get pregnant, give birth safely, and raise the next generation of strong, vibrant children. I deeply, truly hope that this is the path your life follows because I know that's what you want. That's why you are here reading this book.

If you follow the Fertility Fast Track program, the most likely outcome for you is a healthy pregnancy, birth, and baby. But, for a few women, it won't happen this way.

If this is not how your story plays out, I hope that you continue to strive for love, joy, and happiness living a life that may not be your first choice but that still may be more wonderful and fulfilling than you could ever imagine. Among my patients who experience persistent infertility, some choose adoption and some choose to create a life without children. There are no right or wrong answers, only choices.

Over the years, I have been awed and humbled by the strength, determination, and grace I have been privileged to witness in my patients as they confront medical and emotional upheaval. Infertility is a special challenge because it so intimately touches identity.

During my own struggles with infertility, I asked myself, "Who am I as a woman if I can't have children?" Isn't that what the female body is supposed to do? My own body felt empty. Despite how much I loved my husband, my family felt incomplete. I couldn't imagine a childless life.

I was fortunate. My PCOS is relatively mild and I responded to fertility treatments. I got pregnant and I now have four children.

But a very few of my patients have such complex medical situations that despite everything, they don't get pregnant. And I want you to know that they still turn out okay. Some adopt and some don't. Some take a break and try again later. They all find other paths in life. And for some of them, a baby does arrive, unexpectedly, several years down the road. Life is like that.

Women are strong and resilient. Happiness comes in more shapes, colors, and textures than any one of us can imagine.

More than anything, I want to leave you with a message of hope.

If you have followed this Fertility Fast Track program, you have made an enormous investment in your health and fertility. For most women, this investment will pay off in the form of a bright-eyed baby of their very own. For all women, an investment in health is an investment in the present and the future, no matter what else happens.

Because you are more than your capacity to bear or not bear a child. You are more than biology and reproduction.

You are a woman descended from a long line of strong women. Some way somehow, whether through your own biological children or through the lives of the people around you that you touch, you will pass this strength on to future women. This is what all PCOS women do.

Strength. Survival. Resilience.

Whatever happens next, this is your PCOS legacy and destiny.

BONUS SECTION ON MALE FERTILITY

It takes two to tango

Kelton Tremellen, Professor of Reproductive Medicine,
Flinders University. South Australia

One of the key life events that will trigger a woman with PCOS to seek health assistance is a desire to have children. If she follows her doctor's advice, she will lose weight, improve her diet, exercise more, take supplements and perhaps pharmaceutical medications, and may receive targeted medical therapies, all of which can boost her chances of ovulating and conceiving. However, all of this work and the benefits that come from it will not be enough to create a baby if her partner's sperm quality is poor.

That's where you, the male partner, come in. You may be surprised to know that at least 1 in 20 men has a serious reduction in sperm quality, and male factor infertility plays a significant role in up to half of all cases of infertility.

If you are reading this, then your female partner is embarking on a rigorous program to improve her fertility. It is only right and fair for you to embark on a similar journey to make sure you are producing high quality sperm.

When a man ejaculates, the fluid that comes out of his penis is called semen, and it is comprised of lubricants, fructose that serves as fuel for sperm, and, most importantly, many millions of sperm cells per milliliter. Each sperm has a DNA-containing head, a midsection rich in mitochondria that provides the sperm with energy, and a tail that enables the sperm to swim. When we talk about optimizing male fertility, the primary thing we look at is semen quality, which is measured by several characteristics:

- **Quantity:** Current guidelines are that a man needs to have at least 15 million sperm per milliliter (above 40 million per ejaculate would be considered average) to be naturally fertile. Low sperm count is one of the most common types of male-factor infertility.

- **Movement:** The sperm must be alive and swimming—what's referred to as sperm motility. In a healthy sperm sample, at least 40% of the sperm will move properly.

- **Structure:** The sperm must have a proper form, also known as morphology. A well-formed sperm has a nice, oval head and a long, whiplike tail. In a normal sperm sample, at least 4% will have a healthy morphology.

- **Additional characteristics:** Although sperm quantity and quality are the main drivers of male fertility, there can be other problems with semen. We also look at volume (Do you produce enough semen?), liquification (Is your semen the right consistency to allow sperm to swim properly?), fructose levels (Does your semen have enough fructose to feed your sperm?), and pH level (Is your semen the proper pH level to allow your sperm to survive in the female reproductive tract?)

Here are the seven steps to optimize male fertility potential. These lifestyle changes are fairly straightforward and they are good for your overall health, which you will need if you are hoping to start a family. Additionally, when you take responsibility for your health and fertility, you signal to your partner that you are a team and that neither of you carries more responsibility for healthy reproduction than the other.

The seven steps to sperm health

1. **Maintain a normal weight.** Over two-thirds of adult Americans are overweight or obese. In men, fat tissue can lower your testosterone levels by converting your testosterone into the female hormone, estrogen. This hormonal change, combined with other adverse metabolic effects such as inflammation, cardiovascular disease, and insulin resistance, impairs sexual performance (low libido, erectile function) and sperm health. In general, obese men have lower sperm counts, impaired sperm motility, and significantly higher rates of erectile dysfunction.

   Not surprisingly, rising obesity rates have been linked to a decline in sperm quality and an increase in rates of male-factor infertility.[1]

   If you are overweight, then you need to lose weight in order to improve your fertility. Dr. Gersh's fertility program with its healthy diet, time-restricted eating, periodic fasting on the Fasting Mimicking Diet, and moderate exercise program, is an excellent prescription for healthy weight loss.

2. **Adopt a healthy diet.** Of course, you should avoid high-fat/high-sugar foods, drinks, and snacks that are prone to cause weight gain. But more importantly, men seeking to optimize their sperm health should increase their intake of nutritious, fertility-promoting foods. The core of any healthy diet is large quantities of fresh fruits and vegetables, which are high in natural antioxidants. Nuts (especially walnuts) contain important minerals and nutrients that boost sperm quality. In studies, half a cup of nuts

per day significantly improves sperm count, vitality, motility, and morphology. Furthermore, foods high in anti-inflammatory omega-3 oils, such as oily fish (salmon and the like), also improve sperm health.[2,3]

Conversely, you should avoid eating a diet high in red meat and saturated fat because those foods are pro-inflammatory and harmful to testicular health. Additionally, while the evidence for a detrimental effect is mixed, men should probably avoid eating large amounts of soy products such as tofu because they contain natural plant estrogens.

The diet that Dr. Gersh recommends for your partner to improve her fertility is a nutrient-rich, antioxidant-dense, high-fiber, low-sugar, moderate-fat, overall healthy diet. If you want to support your partner while improving your own fertility, eat what she eats. Just add more nuts and go easy on the soy.

3. **Avoid smoking and minimize alcohol intake.** Smoking has clearly been linked to a reduction in sperm health. Specifically, smoking damages the DNA that each sperm carries, which is the DNA used to make your baby. Damaged DNA reduces the chances of conception and increases the risk of miscarriage. Furthermore, several Chinese studies report that the children of fathers who smoked at the time of conception have significantly higher rates of childhood cancer and congenital heart defects. Finally, if you expose your non-smoking female partner to cigarette smoke (so called "side-stream smoke" or "secondhand smoke"), this will reduce her chances of conceiving during IVF treatment. Consequently, you should totally avoid smoking when trying to conceive. If this isn't possible, smoke as little as possible, smoke outside and away from your partner, and after you finish, change your clothes and wash your hands.[4,5,6]

Nicotine replacement therapy does not harm sperm, so you should strongly consider using these products to help you quit smoking. Just so you know, all nicotine, including smoking cessation products, are bad for pregnant women, so if your female partner is also quitting smoking, she will not be able to use those products once she is pregnant. She will need your unwavering support, encouragement, and help. Under no circumstances should you ever smoke around her.

Alcohol has also been shown to reduce sperm quality, especially when consumed in large, binge amounts. Although your female partner should avoid alcohol entirely, it is probably safe for you to consume one to two drinks of alcohol per day while trying to have a baby. However, alcohol use in excess of this should be avoided. Furthermore, it is unfair for a woman to have to abstain completely from alcohol while trying to conceive, while her man drinks to his heart's content. Show some solidarity, future dad, and ease up on the alcohol!

4. **Take a supplement.** One of the key causes of reduced sperm quality and infertility is oxidative stress (OS). Oxidative stress is the process where the body produces too many damaging free radical chemicals that overcome the protective antioxidant capabilities of your body. Oxidative stress causes chronic inflammation, tissue damage, and premature aging, and it has been identified in up to 70% of men who are in an infertile relationship.[7]

Free radicals damage your sperms' outer membranes, stiffen your sperms' tails, and reduce your sperms' capacity to swim. Furthermore, damage to the sperm head membrane can interfere with sperm-egg fusion and block fertilization. Finally, sperm oxidative stress has been linked with damage (fragmentation) to the sperm DNA—a dangerous process that has been linked with infertility, miscarriage, and even with poor health in any resulting children. As such, it is imperative that all men seeking fertility try to minimize oxidative stress.

Sperm oxidative stress happens when there is an increase in the production of free radical chemicals (as occurs with obesity-related inflammation or smoking) or a decline in protective antioxidants received through diet. Fortunately, men can boost their antioxidant defenses by consuming the fertility promoting foods outlined above (fruits, vegetables, nuts, and oily fish), plus additional antioxidant supplements. While there are a multitude of antioxidant supplements available, try looking for one with a broad range of complementary antioxidants of differing action. I recommend a combination of vitamins C and E, lycopene, coenzyme Q10 (CoQ10), zinc, and selenium. Alpha lipoic acid (ALA) is an excellent antioxidant, and in studies, 600 mg per day for 12 weeks dramatically improves sperm count and sperm motility. If you don't eat much fish, an omega-3 supplement also improves sperm health.[8]

In addition to antioxidant levels, a man's gut microbiome (his intestinal bacteria) can also alter his testicular function. This is an area of particular interest of mine. With my research colleagues, I have developed what is aptly-named the GELDING theory (Gut Endotoxin Leading to a Decline IN Gonadal function). Our studies show that an unhealthy gut microbiome causes intestinal permeability, so-called "leaky gut." This allows gut bacteria and gut endotoxins to cross the intestinal wall and enter your bloodstream, where they cause inflammation, decrease testosterone production, and impair sperm health. There is a robust inverse relationship between endotoxin levels in a man's blood and the amount of testosterone he produces: the more endotoxin, the less testosterone.[9,10]

In response to this, several studies now suggest that supplementing with good bacteria, such as with a lactobacillus probiotic, and combining that with bacteria-friendly foods high in prebiotic fiber, such as fruits, vegetables, and beans, can actually boost a man's testosterone levels and sperm health. While this therapy is still in its infancy, probiotics are an exciting new potential treatment for male infertility. Because of the extremely low risk of adverse side effects, I recommend that all men who are trying to conceive take a daily probiotic.[11,12,13]

5. **Avoid occupational or hobby toxins.** Certain activities can damage your sperm by exposing them to toxic chemicals or excess heat. Heavy metals reduce sperm heath, raise male infertility

rates, and increase the risk of your partner having a miscarriage. Common exposure routes are through welding or soldering or the manufacture of lead acid batteries. If you participate in these activities through your job or hobby, be sure to avoid metal fumes by wearing appropriate protective equipment and working in well-ventilated areas, preferably outside.

Other synthetic chemicals can also damage sperm. Pesticides, herbicides, insecticides, and chemicals found in solvents, such as glycol ethers, all lower sperm count and sperm motility. If you handle industrial chemicals, follow all safety precautions to limit your exposure. This also goes for household chemicals such as degreasers, paints, adhesives, and cleaners.[14]

Heat is bad for sperm as well. The testicles are located outside of the body in the scrotum because this keeps them 2 to 3 degrees Celsius/3 to 5 degrees Fahrenheit cooler than core body temperature. The testicles must be kept at this cooler temperature to produce sperm. Any clothing or activity that heats the testicles will impair sperm production and should be minimized. This includes occupational exposure to heat in blast furnaces, cooking in hot restaurant kitchens, taking long, hot baths or saunas, or working with your laptop on your lap. Furthermore, clothing that holds the testicles tight to the body, such as lycra often worn by cyclists, will also heat the testicles and may result in infertility.

Whenever feasible, wear loose-fitting, cotton boxers and pants so your testicles can hang away from your body and stay cool. Avoid activities that expose your testicles to heat.

6. **Medications.** Some medications can have a negative impact on sperm quality. Treatments used to treat male pattern balding (finasteride) are a common example of pharmaceuticals used by men in the reproductive age group, but these class of drugs interfere with testosterone levels and have been linked with increases in sperm DNA damage. Therefore, if you are on any prescription medications, ask your doctor if they are safe to use while you are trying to conceive.

7. **Do not wait too long!** While the decline in male fertility with increasing age is not as pronounced as that seen in women, it does still occur. Sperm number and motility decline with age, while sperm DNA damage increases. The cumulative effects of male aging cause an increase in male factor infertility, especially in men who are 40 and older. Even more worrying, advanced paternal age beyond 50 has been linked with increased risks of autism, schizophrenia, and some rare genetic disorders, such as dwarfism, in their children. As such, do not wait too long before you begin trying to start your family.[15]

Start taking care of your sperm today. Sperm take approximately 70 days to be produced, so for any lifestyle change you make, it will take at least two and a half months before you see the full benefit. Conversely, any sperm toxicant behavior you engage in (smoking, binge-drinking, chemical exposures, soaking in a hot jacuzzi) can negatively impact your semen quality for a full two and a half months. Producing healthy sperm is an on-going commitment.

If you and your partner have not conceived within 6 to 12 months of trying (12 months for women under 35 years, 6 months for women 35 and older) most doctors suggest that, as a couple, you seek fertility help.

If you end up working with a fertility specialist, you will undergo a semen analysis. It's an inexpensive, risk-free test that provides detailed information on your fertility potential. As your partner undergoes fertility treatments, it is critically important that you continue to maintain a sperm-healthy lifestyle so that every round of assisted reproductive therapy has the best chance possible of being successful and creating a healthy baby.

No matter how you end up building your family, remember that when you make a baby, half of your baby's DNA comes from you. You owe it to your partner and future children to do everything in your power to make the sperm who carry that DNA as healthy as possible. Follow these seven straightforward steps, and help your partner as she embarks on her own fertility-maximizing journey.

Best of luck to you both!

Professor Kelton Tremellen
Bachelor of Medicine with honours, Ph.D., Fellow of the
Royal Australian New Zealand College of Obstetricians and
Gynaecologists (FRANZCOG), and Certified subspecialist in
Reproductive Endocrinology and Infertility (CREI)

Professor Tremellen is a sub-specialist gynaecologist (reproductive
endocrinology and infertility) practicing in Adelaide, South Australia
and Professor of Reproductive Medicine at Flinders University. He has an
active research interest in the fields of male infertility, immune mediated
implantation failure, and the impact of nutrition on reproduction.
Professor Tremellen is an acknowledged expert on the impact of
oxidative stress on male fertility and is the inventor of the male fertility
nutraceutical Menevit marked by Bayer.

Workbook A: Medical care workbook

*U*se these pages to guide your conversations with your doctors and care providers and to track the results of any medical tests.

Preconception appointment overview

Read this section before your preconception visit with your primary care physician, midwife, or OB-GYN. The goal of this appointment is to get a general assessment of your health, discuss birth control options, review any medications you are taking, run blood work, identify any unique pregnancy challenges you might be facing, and get her sign-off that you can safely follow the PCOS SOS Fertility Fast Track program. Here is some background information on the topics you will likely discuss.

General health assessment

Most exams start with a general health assessment. Here are some topics to go over:

- **Weight:** What is a healthy target weight for you? If you are overweight, losing 5% to 10% of your body weight can greatly enhance your chances of getting pregnant. Likewise, if you are underweight, gaining proper weight will increase your fertility. In general, a healthy body mass index (BMI) between 18.5 and 24.9 correlates to optimal female fertility.

- **Blood pressure:** Blood pressure consists of two numbers. The upper number, systolic blood pressure, is the amount of force your blood exerts on your artery walls during a heart beat. The lower number, diastolic blood pressure, is the amount of pressure on your artery walls between heart beats while your heart is filling with blood. In general, lower is better. Healthy blood pressure is less than 120/80. High blood pressure increases your risk of early pregnancy loss and pregnancy complications. If your blood pressure is high, discuss healthy targets with your doctor. page 327 for more information on blood pressure measurements.[1]

- **Menstruation:** Long time spans between menstrual cycles can increase your risk for irregular bleeding and endometrial cancer. If it's been longer than three months since your last menstrual cycle, you should request a treatment with progesterone or a progestin to induce a withdrawal bleed from your uterus. I recommend a 14-day treatment course, but some doctors treat for fewer days.

- **Sleep Apnea:** Discuss whether you should be screened for sleep apnea. This disorder is very common among PCOS women. Sleep apnea disrupts your sleep and increases your risks for mood disorders, cardiovascular disease, diabetes, and infertility.

- **PCOS Diagnosis:** Do you have a formal PCOS diagnosis? If not, please discuss with your doctor. She needs to screen you for certain conditions, such as acquired adrenal hyperplasia and thyroid disorders, that have many of the same symptoms as PCOS.

Birth control options

For the next 12 weeks, you want to experience your natural menstrual rhythms (whatever they are or are not). But you don't want to get pregnant. You will be fasting and taking some supplements that are great for restoring fertility but are not proven safe during pregnancy. Please discuss with your doctor the best way to prevent pregnancy during the 12 weeks of the Fertility Fast Track program.

If you are using any form of chemical or hormonal birth control, you need to stop as soon as possible. This includes birth control pills, all types of intrauterine devices (IUDs), vaginal rings, patches, and implants. If you have an IUD or implant, ask your doctor to remove it.

For my patients who are optimizing their health before getting pregnant, I usually recommend the Fertility Awareness Method (FAM). It will provide you with a deep understanding of your fertility cycle that will later help when you are trying to get pregnant. You can find a nice, medically accurate overview here: www.birth-control-comparison.info/fertility-awareness.

To use FAM contraception, monitor your fertility signs. Abstain from sex on your fertile days and have unprotected sex whenever you want on your infertile days. With a high-quality ovulation tracker (recommendations on page 47), monitoring your fertility is pretty simple. Even so, it's a great idea to discuss physical signs of ovulation with your doctor so you know what to look for.

Condoms are another easy method of birth control that don't affect your natural menstrual cycle. I recommend FAM because it's great practice, but please use condoms or another barrier method as backup, especially if you have sex during your fertile days.

Pharmaceutical and nutraceutical review

You and your doctor should review all medications and supplements that you are currently taking. In many cases, with my own patients, we try to wean off most drugs before pregnancy. In particular, I like to take a look at sleeping pills, pain pills, antidepressants, proton pump inhibitors (PPIs), statins, and metformin. In many cases, these pills can be replaced with much safer supplements and lifestyle interventions. But not always.

Every patient is different, so this is something you should discuss with your doctor.

If you decide to stay on specific medications, you may want to follow up with your doctor at the end of this program to reevaluate whether the symptoms you are treating with prescriptions have improved and whether you might, at that point, explore weaning off those drugs.

Substance abuse screening

If you smoke tobacco, use illegal drugs or marijuana, or if you frequently drink alcohol, please discuss with your doctor and make a plan to quit. In the United States, you are protected by HIPAA and patient confidentiality laws, so you can discuss these topics with your doctor without fear. She cannot report you to the police.

If you are abusing prescription drugs and you continue to do so, your doctor may drop you as a patient, but if you are seeking help, this is unlikely.

Unfortunately, drug use is common. We doctors see it all the time. We want you to get help.

Marijuana abuse, tobacco, opioid medications, and illegal drugs are bad for you, bad for your fertility, and bad for the health of your future babies.

Domestic violence abuse screening

Abuse can be physical, verbal, emotional, or financial.

It is finally becoming common practice for doctors to screen patients to identify those at risk of violence. If you feel unsafe for any reason, please tell your doctor, even if she doesn't ask you.

For many women, a doctor's office is a safe space to ask for help, and your doctor can direct you to appropriate resources.

If you are currently unsafe for any reason, it is not your fault. You do not deserve this. Your number one priority is to get safe now.

At any time, you can call:

The National Domestic Violence Hotline at 1–800–799–7233.

Vaginal screening

In addition to a standard pap smear with HPV testing, which screens for cancer and human papilloma virus, you should request a comprehensive DNA analysis of the vaginal microbial population. I highly recommend getting a DNA analysis over the old-fashioned Gram-stained smear. A comprehensive DNA analysis is not a smear or a culture, but rather it is a highly sophisticated test that can detect the population of lactobacilli (good bacteria) you harbor and identify whether you have any overt pathogens growing in the vaginal canal.

Vaginal infections, such as bacterial vaginosis (BV) and other less commonly tested infectious agents such as mycoplasma and ureaplasma, increase your risk of delivering preterm and having a low birth weight baby.

If your DNA analysis comes back positive, you should treat the infection and screen again at three and six months post-treatment because BV and other vaginal infections have extremely high recurrence rates. Your partner should also be tested and treated if the infection found can be passed back and forth.

A healthy vaginal microbiome is key to fertility optimization and a successful pregnancy. Get tested and treated prior to pregnancy.

Lab work

The tests listed here provide critical information about your overall metabolic and hormonal health and provide insight into your potential pregnancy health risks. These tests also create a picture of your specific version of PCOS so you and your doctor can make informed decisions about your healthcare.

Basic tests

All PCOS women should request these tests before attempting to get pregnant. These tests screen for disorders that are exceptionally common in PCOS women and that, if untreated, can lower your chances of getting pregnant and successfully delivering a healthy baby.

Test	What it shows
Antinuclear Antibody Panel (ANA)	If it is high, it indicates a potential autoimmune disease or an elevated risk for a future autoimmune disease.

Test	What it shows
Basic Hormones: · Estradiol · Total Testosterone · DHEAS · FSH · LH	Can help diagnose PCOS, identify your specific type of PCOS, and provide information on your PCOS severity.
Basic Nutrients: · Ferritin (as a marker for iron levels) · Vitamin D (as a 25 OH Vitamin D test)	Nutrient deficiencies lead to poor health. Iron and vitamin D deficiencies are common, especially among PCOS women. Optimal vitamin D is 40-60 ng/mL.
Complete Blood Count (CBC)	Can identify blood disorders, anemia, and immune system disorders.
Comprehensive Metabolic Panel (CMP), preferred to do fasting	Assessment of overall body health. Can identify underlying metabolic disorders such as kidney or liver disease, and diabetes or prediabetes.
Hemoglobin A1C	This is a screen for diabetes. If you already have a diabetes diagnosis, this test shows how well your blood sugar levels have been controlled over the past 3 months. If A1C comes back abnormal, get a 3 hour glucose tolerance test.
Lipid Panel: · Total cholesterol · LDL (low-density lipoprotein) · HDL (high-density lipoprotein) · ApoA1 · ApoB · Triglycerides	This test assesses the health of your cardiovascular system. High triglycerides can also indicate liver dysfunction or fatty liver disease.
Thyroid Panel: · TSH · Free T4 · Free T3 · Anti TPO · Thyroglobulin antibodies	Thyroid disorders are common among PCOS women, so all PCOS women should be periodically tested. TSH should be below 2 (or 2.5 max) for pregnancy.

Additional tests

I prefer that all PCOS women get these additional tests. PCOS is a whole-body disorder and it can impact organs and systems throughout your body. Specifically, women with more severe presentations of PCOS often have compounding health conditions. Screening for abnormal hormone levels, nutrient deficiencies, and disease markers sooner rather than later allows you to make informed decisions about your healthcare and fertility.

Test	What it shows
Anti-Müllerian Hormone (AMH), especially if you are older than 35	AMH is a marker for ovarian reserve and a low level could indicate that you have fewer viable eggs left in your ovaries. Conversely, abnormally high AMH can play a role in anovulatory infertility.
Genetic carrier screening	I recommend that both partners get screened to identify any recessive disorders that they may be carriers for. Natera provides an excellent screening along with complimentary genetic counseling (www.natera.com/horizon-carrier-screen).
Inflammation panel	The inflammation panel from Cleveland HeartLab (www.clevelandheartlab.com/test-menu) shows how much inflammation and what inflammation processes are occuring in your body. Women with PCOS tend to have chronic inflammation, which impacts progesterone production, ovarian health, and risk of pregnancy complications. High inflammation markers typically signify gut microbiome dysbiosis, which should be healed prior to pregnancy.
Insulin level	Fasting insulin is a highly sensitive test that can identify insulin resistance before you are diabetic or even prediabetic. It is common to only test glucose, but you can have a borderline glucose result with a very high insulin result. A post-meal insulin is also very useful as a guide to show how your body responds to food. Insulin testing should be combined with glucose levels if a 3 hour glucose tolerance test is indicated.

Test	What it shows
Methylenetetrahydrofolate reductase (MTHFR)	MTHFR mutations are common. Women with two copies of a variant for a MTHFR gene (C677T) have higher rates of recurrent miscarriage, which can be successfully treated.[2]
Nutritional deficiencies test	I really like the NutrEval FMV test by Genova (www.gdx.net/product/nutreval-fmv-nutritional-test-blood-urine). It tests for deficiencies of a wide range of critical nutrients that could impact your ability to have a healthy pregnancy and healthy baby. In addition to the nutrients, it assesses heavy metals, certain neurotransmitter metabolites, digestive enzymes, and probiotic levels. You can add on MTHFR.
Omegacheck	Knowing the ratio of omega-6 fats to omega-3s gives you valuable insight into your risk for diabetes and cardiovascular disease, both of which impact your risk for pregnancy complications. The omega 3 component DHA is critical for a baby's brain development and EPA is necessary for mood health. (www.clevelandheartlab.com/tests/omegacheck)
Sex hormone binding globulin (SHBG)	Both a high or low SHBG test result provides critical information. A very low level, common with PCOS, leads to higher amounts of unbound, or free, testosterone, which causes hyperandrogenism. Low SHBG is also associated with high insulin levels and inflammation. Oral contraceptives raise the production of SHBG. Women who have taken oral contraceptives for several years may maintain high levels of SHBG long after discontinuing them. This can result in sexual dysfunction.
Vitamin B12	A number of medical conditions and medications can cause low B12 levels. B12 deficiency can cause infertility or subfertility, anemia, depression, neuropathies, cognitive troubles, and poor detoxification.

If you have already been trying to get pregnant for a while, if you are older than 35, or if you are suffering from a wide range of health conditions, there is a third round of tests that I recommend for women with persistent infertility (see page 269). It would be completely reasonable to request these additional tests now or at any point in your fertility journey.

Be sure to ask for a copy of all test results. If any tests come back abnormal, discuss these results with your doctor and schedule a follow up appointment in three to six months, after the end of the Fertility Fast Track program, to retest.

Preconception appointment organizer

At your appointment, you should take notes. There's a lot to cover and you won't remember everything afterwards.

Bring to your appointment

☐ This book, with Your Health Information filled out (page 314)

☐ Blood pressure cuff for calibration

☐ Cell phone pictures of the bottles of all medications, substances, and supplements that you take.

Note to your doctor

Dear Healthcare Provider,

Your patient is embarking on a rigorous program to improve her overall health and fertility. Please discuss with this patient any concerns you may have regarding her ability to safely participate in this program.

Key elements of this program include, but are not limited to:

- Time-restricted eating and a nightly fast of up to 13 hours
- Plant-heavy, sugar-free, gluten-free diet
- Moderate exercise
- Five-day Fasting Mimicking Diet (For more information, see prolonfmd.com)
- Supplements (For more information, see page 287)
- Natural, non-hormonal contraception during program

This program often induces significant improvements in metabolic and cardiovascular health, blood glucose control, and autoimmunity. If any of the patient's health metrics or lab work are abnormal, I suggest scheduling a follow-up appointment to occur after this program is completed to retest.

If the patient is on medication to control blood pressure or blood glucose, consider monitoring the patient throughout the program to make sure patient isn't over-medicated as her health improves.

If you have questions, concerns, or feedback, please feel free to email me at mail@integrativemgi.com.

Thank you,
Dr. Felice Gersh, M.D.

Your health information

Fill this section out before your appointment.

Menstrual health

My last period was on _____.

I usually get my period every _____ to _____ weeks and it typically lasts _____ days.

List menstrual symptoms and concerns:

Pharmaceuticals, drugs, supplements, and controlled substances

This is a list of all of the medications (prescription, OTC, and supplements) I am taking. Bring a cell picture of each bottle.

Pharmaceutical	Dosage

This is a list of all of the alcohol, marijuana, and illegal substances I have used in the last three months.

Substance	Frequency of use	Last used

General questions and concerns

These are questions and concerns I'd like to discuss:

Health symptoms:

_____

_____

Medication:

_____

_____

Domestic violence or safety:

_____

_____

Fertility:

_____

_____

Additional topics:

_____

_____

Appointment guide

Use this section to take notes during your appointment.

	Current	Target
Weight		
BMI		
Blood pressure		

Exam topics to review

☐ Menstrual frequency, symptoms, and time since last period.

☐ Do I have a PCOS diagnosis?

☐ Should I be tested for sleep apnea?

☐ What are my general health risk factors?

☐ What are my health risk factors for infertility and pregnancy complications?

☐ If I have an IUD or birth control implant, please remove it.

☐ For the next 12 weeks, is there any reason that Fertility Awareness would not be a reasonable contraception option for me?

☐ Let's review all pharmaceuticals I am currently taking. For any of these, can we make a plan to wean off them?

☐ Review substance abuse risks, and if appropriate, resources to help quit.

☐ Domestic abuse screening.

☐ Review the Note to Your Doctor (page 313) and discuss the elements of the Fertility Fast Track program.

☐ The PCOS Fertility Fast Track includes daily overnight fasts of 12 to 13 hours and three rounds of the Fasting Mimicking Diet. Are there any medical reasons that I cannot participate in these fasts?

☐ Here are all of the supplements that the Fertility Fast Track recommends (page 287). Are there any potential drug interactions or health risks that I should consider?

☐ Review my general questions and concerns (page 315).

☐ Get prescription for preconception lab tests (page 319).

My notes

Preconception tests

I'd like to get the following tests:

Vaginal

☐ Pap smear and HPV testing

☐ Vaginal DNA testing for BV and other vaginal pathogens

Basic lab work

☐ ANA

☐ Basic Hormones: Estradiol, Total Testosterone, DHEAS, FSH, LH

☐ Ferritin

☐ 25 OH Vitamin D

☐ CBC

☐ CMP, preferred to do fasting

☐ Hemoglobin A1C

☐ Lipid Panel: Total cholesterol, LDL, HDL, ApoA1, ApoB, Triglycerides

☐ Thyroid Panel: TSH, Free T4, Free T3, Anti TPO, Thyroglobulin antibodies

Additional tests that I may want

- ☐ AMH, esp. if patient is over 35 years of age

- ☐ Genetic carrier screening (www.natera.com/horizon-carrier-screen)

- ☐ Inflammation panel (www.clevelandheartlab.com/test-menu)

- ☐ Insulin level

- ☐ MTHFR

- ☐ Nutritional deficiencies (www.gdx.net/product/nutreval-fmv-nutritional-test-blood-urine)

- ☐ Omegacheck (www.clevelandheartlab.com/tests/omegacheck)

- ☐ SHBG

- ☐ Vitamin B12

For patients who are over 35 years old or who have been struggling with infertility for over a year, consider ordering the additional tests listed on page 269.

Specialist appointment organizer

For any appointments with any specialist healthcare providers, bring the Preconception Appointment Organizer (page 312).

In addition to reviewing your specific health stats, you'll want to discuss any specific fertility concerns regarding the health conditions that this doctor is treating. Additionally, you should review the Fertility Fast Track program and see if your doctor has any concerns regarding any parts of the protocol. Share the Note to Your Doctor on page 313 with her.

Exam topics to review

☐ How does my health condition impact all stages of fertility (conception, pregnancy, birth, and infant health)?

☐ Are the medications I am taking safe for pregnancy? Are there safer options available?

☐ Review the Note to Your Doctor (page 313) and discuss the elements of the Fertility Fast Track program.

☐ The PCOS Fertility Fast Track includes daily overnight fasts of 12 to 13 hours and three rounds of the Fasting Mimicking Diet. Are there any medical reasons that I cannot participate in these fasts?

☐ Here are all of the supplements that the Fertility Fast Track recommends (page 287). Are there any potential drug interactions or health risks that I should consider?

☐ How should I monitor this health condition while I am on the Fertility Fast Track program?

☐ Are there any symptoms I should watch for that would warrant a call to your office?

☐ When should I schedule a follow-up appointment?

My notes

Test results

If any tests from your primary care provider or medical specialists come back abnormal, make a follow-up appointment after you complete the Fertility Fast Track program to retest.

Test	Result	Will retest on

Workbook B: Weekly health metrics workbook

$\mathcal{E}$very week on Sunday, you should take your basic measurements. This will help you monitor your progress. It is certainly fine to take measurements more often, but aim for at least once per week.

Weight

Keep a scale in your bathroom. For best results, weigh yourself in the morning, naked, after you have used the toilet. Weight is not a simple indicator of health. Your blood pressure, blood glucose control, and other metabolic metrics can improve while your weight stays stable. But if you are overweight, in many cases, as you get healthier, you will lose weight.

Body mass index (BMI)

Your BMI is the relationship of your weight to height. The easiest way to calculate it is to find an online calculator. The BMI has gotten some bad press because it doesn't distinguish between muscle mass and body fat so some very fit bodybuilders get categorized as obese. Additionally, it doesn't distinguish between high-risk abdominal fat, called visceral fat, and lower risk fat that accumulates in a woman's butt and thighs.

Despite these limitations, for the vast majority of women, BMI is a simple and useful metric to track.

- Less than 18.5 is underweight.
- Between 18.5 and 24.9 is ideal.
- Between 25 and 29.9 is overweight.
- Over 30 is obese.

Most women are optimally fertile when their BMI is closer to 20, but every woman is different. Discuss with your doctor what a healthy BMI would be for you.

Waist to hip ratio

Your waist to hip ratio measures whether you are carrying extra weight in your belly (dangerous) or in your hips (better). A higher ratio corresponds to a higher risk of a cardiovascular event like a heart attack or stroke.

Using a soft tape measure, find the circumference of your waist just above your belly button line. Then measure your hips at their widest point. Divide your waist by your hips. For example, if your waist is 30 inches and your hips are 36 inches around, your ratio is 30/36=0.83.

- Below 0.8 is low risk.
- 0.8 to 0.89 is moderate risk.
- 0.9 or above is high risk.

Even if you don't lose much weight, as inflammation in your body decreases, you may see a redistribution of fat from your waist to your hips. This is a sign of improving health.

Blood pressure

In the evening around 8PM, measure your blood pressure. Sit in a chair quietly for 10 minutes and then follow the instructions that came with your blood pressure cuff.

Your blood pressure is comprised of two numbers: The top number is your systolic blood pressure and the bottom number is your diastolic blood pressure. For both numbers, lower is better. The cut-offs for hypertension (high blood pressure) were recently revised, so even if you think your blood pressure is okay, you should double check.[3]

Systolic (top number)		Diastolic (bottom number)	
Less than 120	with	Less than 80	is ideal.
120-129	with	Less than 80	is elevated.
130-139	or	80-89	is high, stage 1.
140 and above	or	90 and above	is high, stage 2.
Above 180	or	Above 120	is hypertensive crisis. **Call your doctor right away!**

Weekly tracker

Use this form to track your measurements and monitor changes as you progress through the Fertility Fast Track program.

	Weight	**BMI**	**Waist to Hip Ratio**	**Blood Pressure**
Week 1				
Week 2				
Week 3				
Week 4				
Week 5				
Week 6				
Week 7				
Week 8				
Week 9				
Week 10				
Week 11				
Week 12				

You may also want to track additional symptoms. You should customize this section to reflect the PCOS symptoms that bother you the most. You may want to track acne, hair thickness, blood glucose, insulin use, mood, sleep, and menstrual cycle.

	Symptom notes
Week 1	
Week 2	
Week 3	
Week 4	
Week 5	
Week 6	
Week 7	
Week 8	
Week 9	
Week 10	
Week 11	
Week 12	

APPENDIX A

Menu inspirations

I thought about including a cookbook, but honestly, I'm not a great chef who invents her own recipes. I'm a busy doctor. I either cook things simply, no recipe needed, or I find great recipes online and in my favorite cookbooks.

Actually, my husband does most of the cooking in our home because he is a much better cook than I am, but even so, this is how he cooks. And it's how I recommend you cook as well: Figure out what you want to eat; then go find a good recipe.

Instead of a cookbook, I've included a list of menu inspirations that are easy to conform to my basic dietary recommendations:

- Eat mostly fruits, vegetables, and whole grains.
- Eat beans every day.
- Eat organic, unprocessed soy three to four times per week.
- Limit meat, fat, dairy, and caffeine.
- No added sugar, gluten, alcohol, or highly processed foods.

I've organized these recommendations by meals, but please don't feel like you have to eat breakfast for breakfast and dinner for dinner.

I think it's so interesting that in many cultures, there are breakfast foods that are distinct from lunch foods that are also distinct from dinner foods. Personally, I find this to be limiting, and I think these "rules" often guide us to less healthy food choices—processed cereal and milk for breakfast, sandwiches with bread, cheese, and processed deli meat for lunch, and a large, meat-heavy dinner.

Please feel free to be creative with your meal-planning. If you want to have breakfast for dinner or dinner for breakfast, you should do so. Enjoy!

Breakfast ideas

Every morning should start off with a large, satisfying, nutritious breakfast. Breakfast should be your biggest meal of the day. If you can, make time in the morning to cook.

Here are some of my favorite breakfasts. Every one of these items can be improved by adding a side of beans and an egg, cooked any style.

- Black bean scramble
- Berries and chia seed pudding parfait
- Breakfast tacos
- Buckwheat or quinoa porridge
- Cowboy breakfast (beans, potatoes, and corn, cooked in a cast iron skillet)
- English breakfast (British baked beans (which are much less sweet than American baked beans), turkey sausage, and grilled tomatoes)
- Fried rice with lots of veggies and soybeans (frozen work great) and an egg mixed in at the end
- Fruit salad
- Grilled asparagus with poached eggs
- Huevos rancheros

- Muesli, homemade and sugar-free
- Pan fried greens (even mixed salad greens are great) with a fried egg
- Potato pancakes, latke style, topped with chunky applesauce
- Steel cut oats or other whole grain porridge
- Tofu scramble
- Veggie omelet

Lunch ideas

Lunch is your midday meal. It provides the energy and nutrients to get you to dinner. It should be smaller than breakfast but still bigger than dinner. Feel free to eat any of the breakfast or dinner meal suggestions for lunch. Or eat a salad. That's what I usually do.

Here are a few more ideas that feel a bit more lunch-like.

- Fajitas with corn tortillas
- Falafel
- Hummus and veggies
- Lettuce wraps with grilled chicken, mushrooms, and peppers
- Mason jar salad
- Miso soup with tofu
- Spring rolls with veggies and tofu
- Stuffed avocado
- Tacos with grilled fish and avocado
- Veggie soup

Salad ideas

I recommend a salad-a-day because salads are an unrivaled way of getting a wide variety of greens, fruits, veggies, and nuts into your diet every day. I usually eat my salad as part of dinner, but lunch and even breakfast salads are equally great. Whenever you eat it, a salad-a-day is one of the best dietary changes you can make.

But it's easy to get into a salad rut.

A salad does not have to be a couple of veggies on a pile of greens. Although that's actually my favorite kind, even I like to mix things up on occasion. If you Google "salad variations," you'll find hundreds of exciting alternatives to the standard garden salad. Here are a few of my favorites that will hopefully get you thinking outside the salad bowl.

- Beet salad
- Brussel sprout slaw
- Chicken salad in a lettuce wrap
- Chinese chicken salad
- Cole slaw, with oil and vinegar dressing
- Egg salad in a lettuce wrap
- Gazpacho (I know this is a soup, but it's really just a liquified salad.)
- Greek salad
- Kale, apple, and almond salad
- Quinoa and avocado salad
- Roasted veggie salad
- Seaweed salad
- Taco salad
- Tomato-cucumber salad
- Waldorf salad

Dinner ideas

I think it goes without saying that there are an infinite variety of healthy dinners, especially if you start exploring traditional recipes from around the world. Keep dinner small and meat-light. Here are some of my favorite dinners.

- Chana masala, an Indian chickpea dish
- Chili, vegetarian or with a small amount of ground turkey or beef

- Curry, Indian or Thai
- Dal
- Fajitas
- Grilled tofu or tempeh
- Lentil "meatloaf"
- Split pea soup
- Stir-fried veggies
- Stuffed peppers
- Sushi
- Swiss chard tacos with pan-fried fish
- Tofu curry
- Veggie burger, bean or lentil based in a lettuce wrap
- White bean Italian soup

Simple sides

You don't have to cook fancy side dishes. Here are a few extremely fast and/or easy sides that help you get more fruits, veggies, beans, and grains on your plate.

- Asparagus, Brussels sprouts, broccoli, or cauliflower, broiled
- Carrots, steamed in the Instant Pot
- Fresh fruit, such as berries, grapes, or cherries, in a bowl
- Fresh veggies, such as snap peas, carrots, or cherry tomatoes, in a bowl
- Greens or bok choy, sauteed with garlic and chicken broth
- Mardarin oranges
- Quinoa or other whole grain
- Slice of melon
- Sweet potato, roasted

Desserts

Nature is full of foods that are naturally sweet. We humans evolved to love sweet treats and you shouldn't deprive yourself of the happiness that comes from a little indulgence. Once you've been on the Fertility Fast Track program for several weeks, your tastes will begin to adjust to your new low-sugar diet, and it will take much less sugar to satisfy a sweet craving. Here are a few of my favorite desserts.

- Apples, cored and baked with raisins in the middle
- Banana Vitamix "ice cream"
- Berries
- Chia pudding
- Chocolate dipped banana rolled in peanuts, frozen on a stick
- Dark chocolate covered nuts
- Dark chocolate square (at least 70% dark chocolate, and preferably over 80%)
- Dates
- Fresh fruit, any kind
- Hot chocolate (cocoa powder, milk alternative, and a tiny bit of honey)
- Popsicles made from blended fruit
- Smoothie cake (different fruit smoothie flavors layered in a cake pan and frozen)
- Whipped coconut cream

Beverages

Water is the healthiest drink there is, but sometimes it's nice to drink something with flavor. This is especially true at parties. Here are some fancy, delicious, low-sugar, alcohol-free beverages.

- Coffee
- Hot chocolate
- Lemon-lime mineral water
- Mocktails, but watch the sugar

- Sparkling water
- Tea
- Virgin mimosa (orange juice + lemon sparkling water in a 3:1 ratio)
- Water with a squirt of fresh lemon or lime

APPENDIX B

Professional relationship disclosure

I actively contribute to the PCOS and nutraceutical communities in a variety of ways. As part of this, I have professional relationships with several companies.

I am a salaried consultant for Pure Encapsulations, which is a brand under the umbrella company, Atrium Innovations, a division of Nestle Health Sciences, and for L-Nutra, the company that developed the ProLon fasting mimicking diet.

Part of what I do for these companies is speak at professional conferences, develop webinars, and present research in order to educate my fellow doctors about integrative medical approaches to diseases and how supplements and fasting can aid in treatment. Equally exciting, I get to advise on new products, develop treatment protocols, and participate in research studies. Consequently, I've been able to direct significant energy and attention toward PCOS issues.

With Pure Encapsulations, I've developed an entire set of nutraceutical protocols called PureWoman. These are protocols targeted at integrative physicians and naturopathic doctors to inform their treatment of women with cardiovascular disease, metabolic disease, detoxification needs, PMS, and, of course, PCOS.

With L-Nutra, I've piloted informal observational studies on the impact of the Fasting Mimicking Diet on women with PCOS. And based on early, favorable results, we are now designing a formal study on fasting and the metabolic and hormonal markers in women with PCOS.

There are a few other companies that I frequently collaborate with. I am an educator and speaker for the Cleveland HeartLab, which is owned by Quest Laboratories, and is a clinical laboratory that develops cutting edge biomarker tests with the goal to change the landscape for cardiovascular and inflammatory diseases. I am an educational speaker and webinar lecturer for ZRT Laboratory. And I serve on the medical advisory board of Ubiome.

References

Introduction

1. Melo AS, Ferriani RA, Navarro PA. Treatment of infertility in women with polycystic ovary syndrome: approach to clinical practice. *Clinics (Sao Paulo)*. 2015;70(11):765–769.
2. Krzysztof Katulski, Adam Czyzyk, Agnieszka Podfigurna-Stopa, Andrea R. Genazzani & Blazej Meczekalski (2015) Pregnancy complications in polycystic ovary syndrome patients, *Gynecological Endocrinology*, 31:2, 87–91.
3. Unluturk U, Harmanci A, Kocaefe C, Yildiz BO. The Genetic Basis of the Polycystic Ovary Syndrome: A Literature Review Including Discussion of PPAR-gamma. *PPAR Res.* 2007;2007:49109.
4. Reddy UM, Wapner RJ, Rebar RW, Tasca RJ. Infertility, assisted reproductive technology, and adverse pregnancy outcomes: executive summary of a National Institute of Child Health and Human Development workshop. *Obstet Gynecol* 2007;109:967–77.
5. D.D.M. Braat, J.M. Schutte, R.E. Bernardus, T.M. Mooij, F.E. van Leeuwen, Maternal death related to IVF in the Netherlands 1984–2008, *Human Reproduction*, Volume 25, Issue 7, July 2010, Pages 1782–1786.
6. Jackson RA, Gibson KA, Wu YW, Croughan MS. Perinatal outcomes in singletons following in vitro fertilization: a meta-analysis. *Obstet Gynecol* 2004;103:551–63.

Chapter 1

1. Azziz R, Dumesic DA, Goodarzi MO. Polycystic ovary syndrome: an ancient disorder?. *Fertil Steril.* 2011;95(5):1544–1548.
2. Suhail A.R. Doi, Mona Al-Zaid, Philip A. Towers, Christopher J. Scott, Kamal A.S. Al-Shoumer, Irregular cycles and steroid hormones in polycystic ovary syndrome, *Human Reproduction*, Volume 20, Issue 9, September 2005, Pages 2402–2408.
3. Blumenfeld Z, Kaidar G, Zuckerman-Levin N, Dumin E, Knopf C, Hochberg Z. Cortisol-Metabolizing Enzymes in Polycystic Ovary Syndrome. *Clin Med Insights Reprod Health.* 2016;10:9–13. Published 2016 May 5.
4. M Prelević, G & I Würzburger, M & Balint-Perić, L. (1993). 24-hour serum Cortisol profiles in women with polycystic ovary syndrome. Gynecological endocrinology: the official journal of the International Society of Gynecological Endocrinology. 7. 179-84.
5. Takuji Nishihara, Shu Hashimoto, Keijiro Ito, Yoshiharu Nakaoka, Kazuya Matsumoto, Yoshihiko Hosoi & Yoshiharu Morimoto (2014) Oral melatonin supplementation improves oocyte and embryo quality in women undergoing *in vitro* fertilization-embryo transfer, Gynecological Endocrinology, 30:5, 359-362.

6. N. Shreeve, F. Cagampang, K. Sadek, M. Tolhurst, A. Houldey, C.M. Hill, N. Brook, N. Macklon, Y. Cheong, Poor sleep in PCOS; is melatonin the culprit?, *Human Reproduction*, Volume 28, Issue 5, May 2013, Pages 1348–1353.

Chapter 2

1. Jessica A. Mong, Fiona C. Baker, Megan M. Mahoney, Ketema N. Paul, Michael D. Schwartz, Kazue Semba and Rae Silver. *Journal of Neuroscience.* 9 November 2011, 31 (45) 16107-16116.
2. Goldstein, C.A. & Smith, Y.R. *Curr Sleep Medicine Rep* (2016) 2: 206.
3. Cristiana Araújo Gontijo, Bruna Borges Macedo Cabral, Laura Cristina Tibiletti Balieiro, Gabriela Pereira Teixeira, Walid Makin Fahmy, Yara Cristina de Paiva Maia, Cibele Aparecida Crispim. (2019) Time-related eating patterns and chronotype are associated with diet quality in pregnant women. *Chronobiology International* 36:1, pages 75-84.
4. Cobb CM, Kelly PJ, Williams KB, Babbar S, Angolkar M, Derman RJ. The oral microbiome and adverse pregnancy outcomes. *Int J Womens Health.* 2017;9:551–559. Published 2017 Aug 8.
5. McGregor JA, French JI. Bacterial vaginosis in pregnancy. *Obstet Gynecol Surv* 2000;55(5 suppl 1):1–19.
6. García-Velasco, Juan Antonio et al. What fertility specialists should know about the vaginal microbiome: a review, *Reproductive BioMedicine Online*, Volume 35, Issue 1, 103 - 112.
7. Eleni Kandaraki, Antonis Chatzigeorgiou, Sarantis Livadas, Eleni Palioura, Frangiscos Economou, Michael Koutsilieris, Sotiria Palimeri, Dimitrios Panidis, Evanthia Diamanti-Kandarakis, Endocrine Disruptors and Polycystic Ovary Syndrome (PCOS): Elevated Serum Levels of Bisphenol A in Women with PCOS, *The Journal of Clinical Endocrinology & Metabolism*, Volume 96, Issue 3, 1 March 2011, Pages E480–E484.
8. Marques-Pinto A, Carvalho D. Human infertility: are endocrine disruptors to blame?. *Endocr Connect.* 2013;2(3):R15–R29. Published 2013 Sep 17.
9. Mallozzi, M. , Bordi, G. , Garo, C. and Caserta, D. (2016), The effect of maternal exposure to endocrine disrupting chemicals on fetal and neonatal development: A review on the major concerns. *Birth Defect Res C*, 108: 224-242.
10. Hewlett, Meghan & Chow, Erika & Aschengrau, Ann & Mahalingaiah, Shruthi. (2016). Prenatal Exposure to Endocrine Disruptors: A Developmental Etiology for Polycystic Ovary Syndrome. *Reproductive Sciences.* 24.
11. Verma, P., K Sharma, A., Shankar, H. et al. *Biol Trace Elem Res* (2018) 184: 325.
12. C.D. Lynch, R. Sundaram, J.M. Maisog, A.M. Sweeney, G.M. Buck Louis, Preconception stress increases the risk of infertility: results from a couple-based prospective cohort study—the LIFE study, *Human Reproduction*, Volume 29, Issue 5, May 2014, Pages 1067–1075.
13. Joel Goh, Jeffrey Pfeffer, and Stefanos Zenios. Exposure To Harmful Workplace Practices Could Account For Inequality In Life Spans Across Different Demographic Groups, *Health Affairs* 2015 34:10, 1761-1768.

Chapter 3

1. Dai H, Milkman KL, Riis J. Put Your Imperfections Behind You: Temporal Landmarks Spur Goal Initiation When They Signal New Beginnings. *Psychol Sci.* 2015;26(12):1927–1936.
2. Björkman, Lars & Lygre, Gunvor & Haug, Kjell & Skjaerven, Rolv. (2018). Perinatal death and exposure to dental amalgam fillings during pregnancy in the population-based MoBa cohort. PLOS ONE. 13. e0208803.
3. Saini R, Saini S, Saini SR. Periodontitis: A risk for delivery of premature labor and low-birth-weight infants. *J Nat Sci Biol Med.* 2010;1(1):40–42.
4. Wang EY, Huang Y, Du QY, Yao GD, Sun YP. Body mass index effects sperm quality: a retrospective study in Northern China. *Asian J Androl.* 2017;19(2):234–237.
5. Yueshan Hu, Erik A. Ehli, Julie Kittelsrud, Patrick J. Ronan, Karen Munger, Terry Downey, Krista Bohlen, Leah Callahan, Vicki Munson, Mike Jahnke, Lindsey L. Marshall, Kelly Nelson, Patricia Huizenga, Ryan Hansen, Timothy J. Soundy, Gareth E. Davies. Lipid-lowering effect of berberine in human subjects and rats, *Phytomedicine*, Volume 19, Issue 10, 2012, Pages 861-867.
6. Li, Yan & Kuang, Hongying & Shen, Wenjuan & Ma, Hongli & Zhang, Yuehui & Stener-Victorin, Elisabet & Hung, Ernest & Ng, Yu & Liu, Jianping & Kuang, Haixue & Hou, Lihui & Wu, Xiao-Ke. (2013). Letrozole, berberine, or their combination for anovulatory infertility in women with polycystic ovary syndrome: Study design of a doubleblind randomised controlled trial. BMJ open. 3. e003934.
7. An, Y. , Sun, Z. , Zhang, Y. , Liu, B. , Guan, Y. and Lu, M. (2014), The use of berberine for women with polycystic ovary syndrome undergoing IVF treatment. *Clin Endocrinol*, 80: 425-431.
8. Chan E: Displacement of Bilirubin from Albumin by Berberine. Neonatology 1993; 63:201-208.
9. Rahmani, A. H., Alsahli, M. A., Aly, S. M., Khan, M. A., & Aldebasi, Y. H. (2018). Role of Curcumin in Disease Prevention and Treatment. *Advanced biomedical research*, 7, 38.

10. Alessandro Pacchiarotti, Gianfranco Carlomagno, Gabriele Antonini & Arianna Pacchiarotti (2016)Effect of myo-inositol and melatonin versus myo-inositol, in a randomized controlled trial, for improving *in vitro* fertilization of patients with polycystic ovarian syndrome, *Gynecological Endocrinology*, 32:1, 69-73.

11. Pedro-Antonio Regidor and Adolf Eduard Schindler, "Myoinositol as a Safe and Alternative Approach in the Treatment of Infertile PCOS Women: A German Observational Study," *International Journal of Endocrinology*, vol. 2016, Article ID 9537632, 5 pages, 2016.

12. Unfer, V., Facchinetti, F., Orrù, B., Giordani, B., & Nestler, J. (2017). Myo-inositol effects in women with PCOS: a meta-analysis of randomized controlled trials. *Endocrine connections*, 6(8), 647-658.

13. R. D'Anna, V. Di Benedetto, P. Rizzo, E. Raffone, M. L. Interdonato, F. Corrado & A. Di Benedetto(2012) Myo-inositol may prevent gestational diabetes in PCOS women, *Gynecological Endocrinology*, 28:6, 440-442.

14. Cheraghi, E., Soleimani Mehranjani, M., Shariatzadeh, S., Nasr Esfahani, M. H., & Alani, B. (2017). N-Acetylcysteine Compared to Metformin, Improves The Expression Profile of Growth Differentiation Factor-9 and Receptor Tyrosine Kinase c-Kit in The Oocytes of Patients with Polycystic Ovarian Syndrome. *International journal of fertility & sterility*, 11(4), 270-278.

15. Thakker, D., Raval, A., Patel, I., & Walia, R. (2015). N-acetylcysteine for polycystic ovary syndrome: a systematic review and meta-analysis of randomized controlled clinical trials. *Obstetrics and gynecology international*, 2015, 817849.

16. Khoshbaten, M., Aliasgarzadeh, A., Masnadi, K., Tarzamani, M. K., Farhang, S., Babaei, H., Kiani, J., Zaare, M., ... Najafipoor, F. (2010). N-acetylcysteine improves liver function in patients with non-alcoholic Fatty liver disease. *Hepatitis monthly*, 10(1), 12-6.

17. Yamamoto, M., Feigenbaum, S. L., Crites, Y., Escobar, G. J., Yang, J., Ferrara, A., & Lo, J. C. (2012). Risk of preterm delivery in non-diabetic women with polycystic ovarian syndrome. *Journal of perinatology: official journal of the California Perinatal Association*, 32(10), 770-6.

18. Y -H Chiu, A E Karmon, A J Gaskins, M Arvizu, P L Williams, I Souter, B R Rueda, R Hauser, J E Chavarro, for the EARTH Study Team, Serum omega-3 fatty acids and treatment outcomes among women undergoing assisted reproduction, *Human Reproduction*, Volume 33, Issue 1, January 2018, Pages 156–165.

19. Olsen, S. , Sorensen, J. , Secher, N. , Hedegaard, M. , Henriksen, T. , Hansen, H. and Grant, A. (1992). Randomised controlled trial of effect of fish-oil supplementation on pregnancy duration. *International Journal of Gynecology & Obstetrics*, 39: 365-366.

20. Aragon, G., Graham, D. B., Borum, M., & Doman, D. B. (2010). Probiotic therapy for irritable bowel syndrome. *Gastroenterology & hepatology*, 6(1), 39-44.

21. Karamali, M., Eghbalpour, S., Rajabi, S., Jamilian, M., Bahmani, F., Tajabadi-Ebrahimi, M., Keneshlou, F., Mirhashemi, SM., Chamani, M., Hashem Gelougerdi, S., Asemi, Z. (2018). Effects of Probiotic Supplementation on Hormonal Profiles, Biomarkers of Inflammation and Oxidative Stress in Women With Polycystic Ovary Syndrome: A Randomized, Double-Blind, Placebo-Controlled Trial. *Arch Iran Med.* 2018 Jan 1;21(1):1-7.

22. Wallace, C., & Milev, R. (2017). The effects of probiotics on depressive symptoms in humans: a systematic review. *Annals of general psychiatry*, 16, 14.

23. Nordqvist M, Jacobsson B, Brantsæter A, et al. Timing of probiotic milk consumption during pregnancy and effects on the incidence of preeclampsia and preterm delivery: a prospective observational cohort study in Norway. *BMJ Open* 2018;8:e018021.

24. Wang, Z., Zhai, D., Zhang, D., Bai, L., Yao, R., Yu, J., ... Yu, C. (2017). Quercetin Decreases Insulin Resistance in a Polycystic Ovary Syndrome Rat Model by Improving Inflammatory Microenvironment. *Reproductive Sciences*, 24(5), 682-690.

25. Rezvan, N., Moini, A., Gorgani-Firuzjaee, S., & Hosseinzadeh-Attar, M. J. (2017). Oral Quercetin Supplementation Enhances Adiponectin Receptor Transcript Expression in Polycystic Ovary Syndrome Patients: A Randomized Placebo-Controlled Double-Blind Clinical Trial. *Cell journal*, 19(4), 627-633.

26. Jahan, S., Abid, A., Khalid, S., Afsar, T., Qurat-Ul-Ain, Shaheen, G., Almajwal, A., Razak, S. (2018). Therapeutic potentials of Quercetin in management of polycystic ovarian syndrome using Letrozole induced rat model: a histological and a biochemical study, *Journal of Ovarian Research*, 11:26.

27. Cribby S, Taylor M, Reid G. Vaginal microbiota and the use of probiotics. *Interdiscip Perspect Infect Dis.* 2008;2008:256490.

28. Fleet, J. C., DeSmet, M., Johnson, R., & Li, Y. (2012). Vitamin D and cancer: a review of molecular mechanisms. *The Biochemical journal*, 441(1), 61-76.

29. Gominak, Stasha & E Stumpf, W. (2012). The world epidemic of sleep disorders is linked to vitamin D deficiency. Medical hypotheses. 79. 132-5.

30. Lin, M. W., & Wu, M. H. (2015). The role of vitamin D in polycystic ovary syndrome. *The Indian journal of medical research*, 142(3), 238-40.

31. Charan, J., Goyal, J. P., Saxena, D., & Yadav, P. (2012). Vitamin D for prevention of respiratory tract infections: A systematic review and meta-analysis. *Journal of pharmacology & pharmacotherapeutics*, 3(4), 300-3.

32. Bretveld RW, Thomas CM, Scheepers PT, Zielhuis GA, Roeleveld N. Pesticide exposure: the hormonal function of the female reproductive system disrupted?. *Reprod Biol Endocrinol.* 2006;4:30. Published 2006 May 31.

Chapter 4

1. Sutton EF, Beyl R, Early KS, Cefalu WT, Ravussin E, Peterson CM. Early Time-Restricted Feeding Improves Insulin Sensitivity, Blood Pressure, and Oxidative Stress Even without Weight Loss in Men with Prediabetes. *Cell Metab.* 2018;27(6):1212–1221.e3.
2. Wilkinson, Michael & Manoogian, Emily & Zadourian, Adena & Lo, Hannah & Panda, Satchidananda & Taub, Pam. (2019). Time-restricted Eating Promotes Weight Loss and Lowers Blood Pressure in Patients with Metabolic Syndrome. *Journal of the American College of Cardiology.* 73. 1843.
3. Loy SL, Chan JK, Wee PH, et al. Maternal Circadian Eating Time and Frequency Are Associated with Blood Glucose Concentrations during Pregnancy. *J Nutr.* 2017;147(1):70–77.
4. Sutton EF, Beyl R, Early KS, Cefalu WT, Ravussin E, Peterson CM. Early Time-Restricted Feeding Improves Insulin Sensitivity, Blood Pressure, and Oxidative Stress Even without Weight Loss in Men with Prediabetes. *Cell Metab.* 2018;27(6):1212–1221.e3.
5. Mörlin, Birgitta & Hammarström, Margareta. (2005). Nitric oxide increases endocervical secretion at the ovulatory phase in the female. *Acta obstetricia et gynecologica Scandinavica.* 84. 883-6.
6. Meher, S., & Duley, L. (2007). Nitric oxide for preventing pre-eclampsia and its complications. *The Cochrane database of systematic reviews, 2,* CD006490.
7. Jelodar G, Masoomi S, Rahmanifar F. Hydroalcoholic extract of flaxseed improves polycystic ovary syndrome in a rat model. *Iran J Basic Med Sci.* 2018;21(6):645–650.
8. W R Phipps, M C Martini, J W Lampe, J L Slavin, M S Kurzer, Effect of flax seed ingestion on the menstrual cycle, *The Journal of Clinical Endocrinology & Metabolism,* Volume 77, Issue 5, 1 November 1993, Pages 1215–1219.

Chapter 5

1. Rachel Leproult, Egidio F. Colecchia, Mireille L'Hermite-Balériaux, Eve Van Cauter; Transition from Dim to Bright Light in the Morning Induces an Immediate Elevation of Cortisol Levels, *The Journal of Clinical Endocrinology & Metabolism,* Volume 86, Issue 1, 1 January 2001, Pages 151–157.
2. Ivy N. Cheung, Phyllis C. Zee, Dov Shalman, Roneil G. Malkani, Joseph Kang, Kathryn J. Reid. Morning and Evening Blue-Enriched Light Exposure Alters Metabolic Function in Normal Weight Adults. PLOS ONE, 2016; 11 (5): e0155601
3. Reid KJ, Santostasi G, Baron KG, Wilson J, Kang J, Zee PC (2014) Timing and Intensity of Light Correlate with Body Weight in Adults. PLoS ONE 9(4): e92251.
4. J Burgess, Helen & F Fogg, Louis & Young, Michael & Eastman, Charmane. (2004). Bright Light Therapy for Winter Depression—Is Phase Advancing Beneficial?. *Chronobiology International.* 21. 759-75.
5. Figueiro, Mariana G. et al., The impact of daytime light exposures on sleep and mood in office workers. *Sleep Health: Journal of the National Sleep Foundation,* Volume 3, Issue 3, 204 - 215.
6. Vandekerckhove F, Van der Veken H, Tilleman K, et al. Seasons in the sun: the impact on IVF results one month later. *Facts Views Vis Obgyn.* 2016;8(2):75–83.
7. Kojima D, Mori S, Torii M, Wada A, Morishita R, Fukada Y. UV-sensitive photoreceptor protein OPN5 in humans and mice. *PLoS One.* 2011;6(10):e26388.
8. Takasu, N.N., Nakamura, T.J., Tokuda, I.T., Todo, T., Block, G.D., & Nakamura, W. (2015). Recovery from Age-Related Infertility under Environmental Light-Dark Cycles Adjusted to the Intrinsic Circadian Period. *Cell reports, 12* 9, 1407-13 .
9. Figueiro, M. G., & Rea, M. S. (2012). Preliminary evidence that light through the eyelids can suppress melatonin and phase shift dim light melatonin onset. *BMC research notes, 5,* 221.
10. I Mason, D Grimaldi, R G Malkani, K J Reid, P C Zee; 0117 Impact of Light Exposure during Sleep on Cardiometabolic Function, *Sleep,* Volume 41, Issue suppl_1, 27 April 2018, Pages A46.
11. Mariana G. Figueiro and Mark S. Rea, "The Effects of Red and Blue Lights on Circadian Variations in Cortisol, Alpha Amylase, and Melatonin," International Journal of Endocrinology, vol. 2010, Article ID 829351, 9 pages, 2010.
12. Kopcso, Krisztina and Lang, Andras. Nighttime Fears of Adolescents and Young Adults. November 03, 2017. Available from: http://www.smgebooks.com/anxiety-disorders/chapters/ANXD-17-03.pdf
13. Higgins JA. Whole grains, legumes, and the subsequent meal effect: implications for blood glucose control and the role of fermentation. *J Nutr Metab.* 2012;2012:829238.
14. Chavarro JE, Rich-Edwards JW, Rosner BA, Willett WC. Protein intake and ovulatory infertility. *Am J Obstet Gynecol.* 2008;198(2):210.e1–210.e2107.

Chapter 6

1. Gamble KL, Resuehr D, Johnson CH. Shift work and circadian dysregulation of reproduction. *Front Endocrinol (Lausanne)*. 2013;4:92. Published 2013 Aug 7.
2. Lim AJ, Huang Z, Chua SE, Kramer MS, Yong EL. Sleep Duration, Exercise, Shift Work and Polycystic Ovarian Syndrome-Related Outcomes in a Healthy Population: A Cross-Sectional Study. *PLoS One*. 2016;11(11):e0167048. Published 2016 Nov 21.
3. Brum MC, Filho FF, Schnorr CC, Bottega GB, Rodrigues TC. Shift work and its association with metabolic disorders. *Diabetol Metab Syndr*. 2015;7:45. Published 2015 May 17.
4. Fernando S, Rombauts L. Melatonin: shedding light on infertility?--A review of the recent literature. *J Ovarian Res*. 2014;7:98. Published 2014 Oct 21.
5. L.J. Moran, W.A. March, M.J. Whitrow, L.C. Giles, M.J. Davies, V.M. Moore; Sleep disturbances in a community-based sample of women with polycystic ovary syndrome, *Human Reproduction*, Volume 30, Issue 2, 1 February 2015, Pages 466–472.
6. Fernandez, R. C., Moore, V. M., Van Ryswyk, E. M., Varcoe, T. J., Rodgers, R. J., March, W. A., Moran, L. J., Avery, J. C., McEvoy, R. D., ... Davies, M. J. (2018). Sleep disturbances in women with polycystic ovary syndrome: prevalence, pathophysiology, impact and management strategies. *Nature and science of sleep*, 10, 45–64.
7. Alexandros N. Vgontzas, Richard S. Legro, Edward O. Bixler, Allison Grayev, Anthony Kales, George P. Chrousos, Polycystic Ovary Syndrome Is Associated with Obstructive Sleep Apnea and Daytime Sleepiness: Role of Insulin Resistance, *The Journal of Clinical Endocrinology & Metabolism*, Volume 86, Issue 2, 1 February 2001, Pages 517–520.
8. Macrea, M.M., Martin, T.J., & Zăgrean, L. (2010). Infertility and obstructive sleep apnea: the effect of continuous positive airway pressure therapy on serum prolactin levels. *Sleep and Breathing*, 14, 253-257.
9. Koopman, A., Rauh, S. P., van 't Riet, E., Groeneveld, L., van der Heijden, A. A., Elders, P. J., Dekker, J. M., Nijpels, G., Beulens, J. W., ... Rutters, F. (2017). The Association between Social Jetlag, the Metabolic Syndrome, and Type 2 Diabetes Mellitus in the General Population: The New Hoorn Study. *Journal of biological rhythms*, 32(4), 359-368.
10. Jain, P., Jain, M., Haldar, C., Singh, T. B., & Jain, S. (2013). Melatonin and its correlation with testosterone in polycystic ovarian syndrome. *Journal of human reproductive sciences*, 6(4), 253-8.
11. Ferracioli-Oda E, Qawasmi A, Bloch MH (2013) Meta-Analysis: Melatonin for the Treatment of Primary Sleep Disorders. *PLoS ONE* 8(5): e63773.
12. Rai, Seema & Basheer, Muddasir. (2015). Melatonin Attenuates Free Radical Load and Reverses Histologic Architect and Hormone Profile Alteration in Female Rat: An In vivo Study of Pathogenesis of Letrozole Induced Poly Cystic Ovary. *Journal of Clinical & Cellular Immunology*. 06.
13. Alessandro Pacchiarotti, Gianfranco Carlomagno, Gabriele Antonini & Arianna Pacchiarotti (2016)Effect of myo-inositol and melatonin versus myo-inositol, in a randomized controlled trial, for improving in vitro fertilization of patients with polycystic ovarian syndrome, *Gynecological Endocrinology*, 32:1, 69-73.
14. Tagliaferri, Valeria & Romualdi, Daniela & Scarinci, Elisa & De Cicco, Simona & Di Florio, Christian & Immediata, Valentina & Tropea, Anna & Mariaflavia Santarsiero, Carla & Lanzone, Antonio & Apa, Rosanna. (2017). Melatonin Treatment May Be Able to Restore Menstrual Cyclicity in Women With PCOS: A Pilot Study. *Reproductive Sciences*. 25. 193371911771126.
15. Vittorio Unfer, Emanuela Raffone, Piero Rizzo & Silvia Buffo (2011) Effect of a supplementation with myo-inositol plus melatonin on oocyte quality in women who failed to conceive in previous in vitro fertilization cycles for poor oocyte quality: a prospective, longitudinal, cohort study, *Gynecological Endocrinology*, 27:11, 857-861.
16. Zizhen Xie, Fei Chen, William A. Li, Xiaokun Geng, Changhong Li, Xiaomei Meng, Yan Feng, Wei Liu & Fengchun Yu (2017) A review of sleep disorders and melatonin, *Neurological Research*, 39:6, 559-565.
17. Silman, R.E., Melatonin: a contraceptive for the nineties. *European Journal of Obstetrics & Gynecology*, Volume 49, Issue 1, 3 - 9.
18. Herxheimer A, Petrie KJ. Melatonin for the prevention and treatment of jet lag. *Cochrane Database of Systematic Reviews* 2002, Issue 2. Art. No.: CD001520.
19. Jun Yoshino, Paloma Almeda-Valdes, Bruce W. Patterson, Adewole L. Okunade, Shin-ichiro Imai, Bettina Mittendorfer, Samuel Klein, Diurnal Variation in Insulin Sensitivity of Glucose Metabolism Is Associated With Diurnal Variations in Whole-Body and Cellular Fatty Acid Metabolism in Metabolically Normal Women, *The Journal of Clinical Endocrinology & Metabolism*, Volume 99, Issue 9, 1 September 2014, Pages E1666–E1670.
20. Jakubowicz, D., Barnea, M., Wainstein, J. and Froy, O. (2013), High Caloric intake at breakfast vs. dinner differentially influences weight loss of overweight and obese women. *Obesity*, 21: 2504-2512.
21. Daniela Jakubowicz, Maayan Barnea, Julio Wainstein, Oren Froy. Effects of caloric intake timing on insulin resistance and hyperandrogenism in lean women with polycystic ovary syndrome. *Clinical Science*, 2013; 125 (9): 423.

22. Marinac CR, Sears DD, Natarajan L, Gallo LC, Breen CI, Patterson RE. Frequency and Circadian Timing of Eating May Influence Biomarkers of Inflammation and Insulin Resistance Associated with Breast Cancer Risk. PLoS One. 2015 Aug 25;10(8):e0136240.

Chapter 7

1.   Kandaraki, Eleni & Chatzigeorgiou, Antonios & Livadas, Sarantis & Palioura, Eleni & Economou, Frangiscos & Koutsilieris, Michael & Palimeri, Sotiria & Panidis, Dimitrios & Diamanti-Kandarakis, Evanthia. (2010). Endocrine Disruptors and Polycystic Ovary Syndrome (PCOS): Elevated Serum Levels of Bisphenol A in Women with PCOS. The Journal of clinical endocrinology and metabolism. 96. E480-4.
2.   Do, M. T., Chang, V. C., Mendez, M. A., & de Groh, M. (2017). Urinary bisphenol A and obesity in adults: results from the Canadian Health Measures Survey Concentration urinaire de bisphénol A et obésité chez les adultes : résultats de l'Enquête canadienne sur les mesures de la santé. Health promotion and chronic disease prevention in Canada : research, policy and practice, 37(12), 403-412.
3.   G Boucher, Jonathan & Boudreau, Adèle & Ahmed, Shaimaa & Atlas, Ella. (2015). In Vitro Effects of Bisphenol A β-D-Glucuronide (BPA-G) on Adipogenesis in Human and Murine Preadipocytes. Environmental health perspectives. 123.
4.   Hwang S, Lim JE, Choi Y, Jee SH. Bisphenol A exposure and type 2 diabetes mellitus risk: a meta-analysis. BMC Endocr Disord. 2018;18(1):81. Published 2018 Nov 6.
5.   Ziv-Gal A, Flaws JA. Evidence for bisphenol A-induced female infertility: a review (2007-2016). Fertil Steril. 2016;106(4):827–856.
6.   Huo X, Chen D, He Y, Zhu W, Zhou W, Zhang J. Bisphenol-A and Female Infertility: A Possible Role of Gene-Environment Interactions. Int J Environ Res Public Health. 2015;12(9):11101–11116. Published 2015 Sep 7.
7.   The Endocrine Society. "BPA exposure during pregnancy can alter circadian rhythms." ScienceDaily. ScienceDaily, 25 March 2019.
8.   Fischer, C.P., Mamillapalli, R., Goetz, L.G., Jorgenson, E., Ilagan, Y., & Taylor, H.S. (2016). Bisphenol A (BPA) Exposure In Utero Leads to Immunoregulatory Cytokine Dysregulation in the Mouse Mammary Gland: A Potential Mechanism Programming Breast Cancer Risk. Hormones and Cancer, 7, 241-251.
9.   Klenke, U., & Hutchins, B. I. (2011). Using bisphenol-a to study the onset of polycystic ovarian syndrome. Frontiers in endocrinology, 2, 12.
10. Rutkowska, Aleksandra & Rachoń, Dominik. (2014). Bisphenol A (BPA) and its potential role in the pathogenesis of the polycystic ovary syndrome (PCOS). Gynecological endocrinology : the official journal of the International Society of Gynecological Endocrinology. 30.
11. Rashidi, B.H., Amanlou, M., Lak, T.B., Ghazizadeh, M., Haghollahi, F., Bagheri, M., & Eslami, B. (2017). The Association Between Bisphenol A and Polycystic Ovarian Syndrome: A Case-Control Study. Acta medica Iranica, 55 12, 759-764 .
12. Monaco, Kristen. (2018, February 13) Nonstick Chemicals May Disrupt Metabolic Function in Women. MedPage Today. Retrieved November 7, 2018 from www.medpagetoday.com/publichealthpolicy/environmentalhealth/71128
13. Centers for Disease Control and Prevention, Water Fluoridation Data & Statistics. Accessed on August 6, 2019. Available from https://www.cdc.gov/fluoridation/statistics/index.htm.
14. Iheozor-Ejiofor Z, Worthington HV, Walsh T, O'Malley L, Clarkson JE, Macey R, Alam R, Tugwell P, Welch V, Glenny AM. Water fluoridation for the prevention of dental caries. Cochrane Database of Systematic Reviews 2015, Issue 6. Art. No.: CD010856.
15. Kumar N, Sood S, Arora B, Singh M, Beena. Effect of duration of fluoride exposure on the reproductive system in male rabbits. J Hum Reprod Sci. 2010;3(3):148–152.
16. Yongjiang Zhou, Yiwen Qiu, Junlin He, Xuemei Chen, Yubing Ding, Yingxiong Wang, Xueqing Liu. The toxicity mechanism of sodium fluoride on fertility in female rats, Food and Chemical Toxicology, Volume 62, 2013, Pages 566-572, ISSN 0278-6915.
17. Małgorzata Szczuko, Joanna Splinter, Marta Zapałowska-Chwyć, Maciej Ziętek, Dominika Maciejewska. Fluorine may intensify the mechanisms of polycystic ovary syndrome (PCOS) development via increased insulin resistance and disturbed thyroid-stimulating hormone (TSH) synthesis even at reference levels, Medical Hypotheses, Volume 128, 2019, Pages 58-63, ISSN 0306-9877.
18. Stan C. Freni (1994) Exposure to high fluoride concentrations in drinking water is associated with decreased birth rates, Journal of Toxicology and Environmental Health, 42:1, 109-121.
19. Sasada T, Hinoi T, Saito Y, Adachi T, Takakura Y, Kawaguchi Y, et al. (2015) Chlorinated Water Modulates the Development of Colorectal Tumors with Chromosomal Instability and Gut Microbiota in Apc-Deficient Mice. PLoS ONE 10(7): e0132435.
20. Kieran D. Cox, Garth A. Covernton, Hailey L. Davies, John F. Dower, Francis Juanes, and Sarah E. Dudas. Human Consumption of Microplastics, Environmental Science & Technology. 2019 53 (12), 7068-7074.

21. Majd, Sanaz (2015, October 21) Should You Drink Tap or Bottled Water? *Scientific American.* Retrieved from: https://www.scientificamerican.com/article/should-you-drink-tap-or-bottled-water/
22. Walker, Mark & Seiler, Ralph & Meinert, Michael. (2008). Effectiveness of household reverse-osmosis systems in a Western US region with high arsenic in groundwater. *The Science of the total environment.* 389. 245-52.

Chapter 8

1. Colberg, Sheri R. et al., Exercise Effects on Postprandial Glycemia, Mood, and Sympathovagal Balance in Type 2 Diabetes. *Journal of the American Medical Directors Association,* 2014 Apr; Volume 15, Issue 4, 261 - 266.
2. Lindsey M Russo, Brian W Whitcomb, Sunni L Mumford, Marquis Hawkins, Rose G Radin, Karen C Schliep, Robert M Silver, Neil J Perkins, Keewan Kim, Ukpebo R Omosigho, Daniel L Kuhr, Tiffany L Holland, Lindsey A Sjaarda, Enrique F Schisterman, A prospective study of physical activity and fecundability in women with a history of pregnancy loss, *Human Reproduction,* Volume 33, Issue 7, July 2018, Pages 1291–1298.
3. Wise LA, Rothman KJ, Mikkelsen EM, Sørensen HT, Riis AH, Hatch EE. A prospective cohort study of physical activity and time to pregnancy. *Fertil Steril.* 2012;97(5):1136–42.e424.
4. D Hall, Kevin. (2019). Ultra-processed diets cause excess calorie intake and weight gain: A one-month inpatient randomized controlled trial of ad libitum food intake. *Cell Metabolism.* 30, 67–77.
5. Jessica A Grieger, Luke E Grzeskowiak, Tina Bianco-Miotto, Tanja Jankovic-Karasoulos, Lisa J Moran, Rebecca L Wilson, Shalem Y Leemaqz, Lucilla Poston, Lesley McCowan, Louise C Kenny, Jenny Myers, James J Walker, Robert J Norman, Gus A Dekker, Claire T Roberts, Pre-pregnancy fast food and fruit intake is associated with time to pregnancy, *Human Reproduction,* Volume 33, Issue 6, June 2018, Pages 1063–1070.
6. Hatch EE, Wesselink AK, Hahn KA, et al. Intake of Sugar-sweetened Beverages and Fecundability in a North American Preconception Cohort. *Epidemiology.* 2018;29(3):369–378.
7. Collin LJ, Judd S, Safford M, Vaccarino V, Welsh JA. Association of Sugary Beverage Consumption With Mortality Risk in US Adults: A Secondary Analysis of Data From the REGARDS Study. *JAMA Netw Open.* Published online May 17, 20192(5):e193121.
8. Panth N, Gavarkovs A, Tamez M, Mattei J. The Influence of Diet on Fertility and the Implications for Public Health Nutrition in the United States. *Front Public Health.* 2018;6:211. Published 2018 Jul 31.
9. Afshin, Ashkan & John Sur, Patrick & A. Fay, Kairsten & Cornaby, Leslie & Ferrara, Giannina & S Salama, Joseph & C Mullany, Erin & Abate, Kalkidan & Cristiana, Abbafati & Abebe, Zegeye & Afarideh, Mohsen & Aggarwal, Anju & Agrawal, Sutapa & Akinyemiju, Tomi & Alahdab, Fares & Bacha, Umar & F Bachman, Victoria & Badali, Hamid & Badawi, Alaa. (2019). Health effects of dietary risks in 195 countries, 1990–2017: a systematic analysis for the Global Burden of Disease Study 2017. *The Lancet.* 393. 1958-1972.

Chapter 9

1. Higgins JA. Whole grains, legumes, and the subsequent meal effect: implications for blood glucose control and the role of fermentation. *J Nutr Metab.* 2012;2012:829238.
2. Reverri EJ, Randolph JM, Steinberg FM, Kappagoda CT, Edirisinghe I, Burton-Freeman BM. Black Beans, Fiber, and Antioxidant Capacity Pilot Study: Examination of Whole Foods vs. Functional Components on Postprandial Metabolic, Oxidative Stress, and Inflammation in Adults with Metabolic Syndrome. *Nutrients.* 2015;7(8):6139-6154. Published 2015 Jul 27.
3. Tonstad, S., Malik, N.A., & Haddad, E. (2014). A high-fibre bean-rich diet versus a low-carbohydrate diet for obesity. *Journal of human nutrition and dietetics : the official journal of the British Dietetic Association,* 27 Suppl 2, 109-16 .
4. Ganesan K, Xu B. Polyphenol-Rich Dry Common Beans (Phaseolus vulgaris L.) and Their Health Benefits. *Int J Mol Sci.* 2017;18(11):2331. Published 2017 Nov 4.
5. Winham DM, Hutchins AM. Perceptions of flatulence from bean consumption among adults in 3 feeding studies. *Nutr J.* 2011;10:128. Published 2011 Nov 21.
6. Riitta Törrönen, Marjukka Kolehmainen, Essi Sarkkinen, Hannu Mykkänen, Leo Niskanen, Postprandial glucose, insulin, and free fatty acid responses to sucrose consumed with blackcurrants and lingonberries in healthy women, *The American Journal of Clinical Nutrition,* Volume 96, Issue 3, September 2012, Pages 527–533.
7. Qu, X.M. & Wu, Z.F. & Pang, B.X. & Jin, L.Y. & Qin, L.Z. & Wang, S.L.. (2016). From Nitrate to Nitric Oxide: The Role of Salivary Glands and Oral Bacteria. *Journal of Dental Research.* 95.
8. Ercolini D, Fogliano V. Food Design To Feed the Human Gut Microbiota. *J Agric Food Chem.* 2018;66(15):3754–3758.

9.   Marinac CR, Nelson SH, Breen CI, et al. Prolonged Nightly Fasting and Breast Cancer Prognosis. *JAMA Oncol.* 2016;2(8):1049–1055.
10.   Shuang Rong, Linda G. Snetselaar, Guifeng Xu, Yangbo Sun, Buyun Liu, Robert B. Wallace, Wei Bao. Association of Skipping Breakfast With Cardiovascular and All-Cause Mortality, *Journal of the American College of Cardiology.* Apr 2019, 73 (16) 2025-2032.
11.   Munsters MJ, Saris WH. Effects of meal frequency on metabolic profiles and substrate partitioning in lean healthy males. *PLoS One.* 2012;7(6):e38632.

Chapter 10

1.   Razzoli, M, Nyuyki-Dufe, K, Gurney, A, et al. Social stress shortens lifespan in mice. *Aging Cell.* 2018; 17:e12778.
2.   Stephen E. Gilman, Ewa Sucha, Mila Kingsbury, Nicholas J. Horton, Jane M. Murphy and Ian Colman. Depression and mortality in a longitudinal study: 1952–2011, CMAJ. October 23, 2017, 189 (42) E1304-E1310.
3.   Cantarero-Prieto D, Pascual-Sáez M, Blázquez-Fernández C. Social isolation and multiple chronic diseases after age 50: A European macro-regional analysis. *PLoS One.* 2018;13(10):e0205062. Published 2018 Oct 24.
4.   Patel A, Sharma PS, Narayan P, Binu VS, Dinesh N, Pai PJ. Prevalence and predictors of infertility-specific stress in women diagnosed with primary infertility: A clinic-based study. *J Hum Reprod Sci.* 2016;9(1):28–34.
5.   C.D. Lynch, R. Sundaram, J.M. Maisog, A.M. Sweeney, G.M. Buck Louis, Preconception stress increases the risk of infertility: results from a couple-based prospective cohort study—the LIFE study, *Human Reproduction,* Volume 29, Issue 5, May 2014, Pages 1067–1075.
6.   Tan, J., Wang, Q. Y., Feng, G. M., Li, X. Y., & Huang, W. (2017). Increased Risk of Psychiatric Disorders in Women with Polycystic Ovary Syndrome in Southwest China. *Chinese medical journal,* 130(3), 262-266.
7.   Suzette Bishop, Samuel Basch, and Walter Futterweit (2009) Polycystic Ovary Syndrome, Depression, and Affective Disorders. *Endocrine Practice:* July 2009, Vol. 15, No. 5, pp. 475-482.
8.   Biddle S. Physical activity and mental health: evidence is growing. *World Psychiatry.* 2016;15(2):176–177.
9.   Shohani M, Badfar G, Nasirkandy MP, et al. The Effect of Yoga on Stress, Anxiety, and Depression in Women. *Int J Prev Med.* 2018;9:21. Published 2018 Feb 21.
10.   Nidhi, R.S., Padmalatha, V., Nagarathna, R., & Ram, A. (2012). Effect of a yoga program on glucose metabolism and blood lipid levels in adolescent girls with polycystic ovary syndrome. *International journal of gynaecology and obstetrics: the official organ of the International Federation of Gynaecology and Obstetrics,* 118 1, 37-41.
11.   Rani Monika, Singh Uma, Gopal, A., Madhav, N., Kala Sarswati, Ghildiyal Archana, & Srivastava Neena (2013). Impact of Yoga Nidra on menstrual abnormalities in females of reproductive age, *Journal of Alternative and Complementary Medicine,* Vol. 19, No. 12.
12.   Darbandi, Mahsa & Sara & Khorram Khorshid, Hamid Reza & Sadeghi, Mohammad. (2017). Yoga Can Improve Assisted Reproduction Technology Outcomes in Couples With Infertility. *Alternative therapies in health and medicine.* 24.
13.   Rachel E. Maddux, Daiva Daukantaité & Una Tellhed (2018) The effects of yoga on stress and psychological health among employees: an 8- and 16-week intervention study, *Anxiety, Stress & Coping,* 31:2, 121-134.
14.   Case, L. K., Jackson, P., Kinkel, R., & Mills, P. J. (2018). Guided Imagery Improves Mood, Fatigue, and Quality of Life in Individuals With Multiple Sclerosis: An Exploratory Efficacy Trial of Healing Light Guided Imagery. *Journal of evidence-based integrative medicine,* 23.
15.   Jallo, N., Ruiz, R. J., Elswick, R. K., & French, E. (2014). Guided imagery for stress and symptom management in pregnant african american women. *Evidence-based complementary and alternative medicine : eCAM,* 2014, 840923.
16.   Lee, M. H., Kim, D. H., & Yu, H. S. (2013). The effect of guided imagery on stress and fatigue in patients with thyroid cancer undergoing radioactive iodine therapy. *Evidence-based complementary and alternative medicine : eCAM,* 2013, 130324.
17.   Tammi R.A. Kral, Brianna S. Schuyler, Jeanette A. Mumford, Melissa A. Rosenkranz, Antoine Lutz, Richard J. Davidson. Impact of short- and long-term mindfulness meditation training on amygdala reactivity to emotional stimuli, *NeuroImage,* Volume 181, 2018, Pages 301-313.
18.   Mei-Kei Leung, Way K.W. Lau, Chetwyn C.H. Chan, Samuel S.Y. Wong, Annis L.C. Fung & Tatia M.C. Lee (2018) Meditation-induced neuroplastic changes in amygdala activity during negative affective processing, *Social Neuroscience,* 13:3, 277-288.
19.   Qin, S., Young, C. B., Duan, X., Chen, T., Supekar, K., & Menon, V. (2013). Amygdala subregional structure and intrinsic functional connectivity predicts individual differences in anxiety during early childhood. *Biological psychiatry,* 75(11), 892-900.

20. Gotink, R.A., Vernooij, M.W., Ikram, M.A. et al. Meditation and yoga practice are associated with smaller right amygdala volume: the Rotterdam study, *Brain Imaging and Behavior* (2018).

21. Sina Radke, Inge Volman, Pranjal Mehta, Veerle Van Son, Dorien Enter, Alan Sanfey, Ivan Toni, Ellen R. A. De Bruijn and Karin Roelofs. Testosterone biases the amygdala toward social threat approach. *Science Advances*, 2015.

22. Hölzel, B. K., Carmody, J., Vangel, M., Congleton, C., Yerramsetti, S. M., Gard, T., & Lazar, S. W. (2010). Mindfulness practice leads to increases in regional brain gray matter density. *Psychiatry research*, 191(1), 36-43.

23. Basak Ozgen Saydam, Arzu Ceylan Has, Gurkan Bozdag, Kader Karli Oguz & Bulent Okan Yildiz (2017) Structural imaging of the brain reveals decreased total brain and total gray matter volumes in obese but not in lean women with polycystic ovary syndrome compared to body mass index-matched counterparts, *Gynecological Endocrinology*, 33:7, 519-523.

24. (2013). Effects of odor on emotion, with implications. *Frontiers in systems neuroscience*, 7, 66.

25. Kim, I. H., Kim, C., Seong, K., Hur, M. H., Lim, H. M., & Lee, M. S. (2012). Essential oil inhalation on blood pressure and salivary cortisol levels in prehypertensive and hypertensive subjects. *Evidence-based complementary and alternative medicine: eCAM*, 2012, 984203.

26. Knight, L., A. Levin, AND C. Mendenhall. Candles and Incense as Potential Sources of Indoor Air Pollution: Market Analysis and Literature Review (EPA/600/R-01/001). U.S. *Environmental Protection Agency*, Washington, D.C., 2001.

27. Kim, I. H., Kim, C., Seong, K., Hur, M. H., Lim, H. M., & Lee, M. S. (2012). Essential oil inhalation on blood pressure and salivary cortisol levels in prehypertensive and hypertensive subjects. *Evidence-based complementary and alternative medicine : eCAM*, 2012, 984203.

28. R.P. Silva-Néto, M.F. Peres, M.M. Valença. Odorant substances that trigger headaches in migraine patients, *Cephalalgia*, 34 (2014), pp. 14-21.

29. D. Vethanayagam, H. Vliagoftis, D. Mah, J. Beach, L. Smith, R. Moqbel. Fragrance materials in asthma: a pilot study using a surrogate aerosol product, J *Asthma*, 50 (2013), pp. 975-982.

30. Tiago S. Pavão, Priscila Vianna, Micheli M. Pillat, Amanda B. Machado, Moisés E. Bauer. Acupuncture is effective to attenuate stress and stimulate lymphocyte proliferation in the elderly, *Neuroscience Letters*, Volume 484, Issue 1, 2010, Pages 47-50.

31. Cochrane S, Smith CA, Possamai-Inesedy A, Bensoussan A. Acupuncture and women's health: an overview of the role of acupuncture and its clinical management in women's reproductive health. *Int J Womens Health*. 2014;6:313-325. Published 2014 Mar 17.

32. Cochrane S, Smith CA, Possamai-Inesedy A, Bensoussan A. Prior to Conception: The Role of an Acupuncture Protocol in Improving Women's Reproductive Functioning Assessed by a Pilot Pragmatic Randomised Controlled Trial [published correction appears in Evid Based Complement Alternat Med. 2018 May 2;2018:2343604]. *Evid Based Complement Alternat Med*. 2016;2016:3587569.

33. Campeau, Marie-Pierre & Gaboriault, Réal & Drapeau, Martine & Nguyen, Thu Van & Roy, Indranath & Fortin, Bernard & Marois, Mariette & Nguyen-Tan, P. (2007). Impact of Massage Therapy on Anxiety Levels in Patients Undergoing Radiation Therapy: Randomized Controlled Trial. *Journal of the Society for Integrative Oncology*. 5. 133-8.

34. Sherman, K. J., Ludman, E. J., Cook, A. J., Hawkes, R. J., Roy-Byrne, P. P., Bentley, S. , Brooks, M. Z. and Cherkin, D. C. (2010), Effectiveness of therapeutic massage for generalized anxiety disorder: a randomized controlled trial. *Depress. Anxiety*, 27: 441-450.

Chapter 11

1. Stephen Lester, Michael Schade, Caitlin Weigand. Volatile Vinyl: The New Shower Curtain's Chemical Smell, *Center for Health, Environment and Justice* (CHEJ), June 2008.

2. Kay VR, Chambers C, Foster WG. Reproductive and developmental effects of phthalate diesters in females. *Crit Rev Toxicol*. 2013; 43(3): 200–219.

3. Exposures add up – Survey results, Environmental Working Group. 2004. Available from www.ewg.org/skindeep/2004/06/15/exposures-add-up-survey-results

4. How Much Is Your Face Worth? Our Survey Results Revealed! Skin Store. 2017. Available from www.skinstore.com/blog/skincare/womens-face-worth-survey-2017

5. FDA website, accessed on June 2, 2019. Available from https://www.fda.gov/cosmetics/cosmetics-laws-regulations/fda-authority-over-cosmetics-how-cosmetics-are-not-fda-approved-are-fda-regulated

6. Huang, Po-Chin & Liao, Kai-Wei & Chang, Jung-Wei & Lee, Ching-Chang. (2018). Characterization of phthalates exposure and risk for cosmetics and perfume sales clerks. *Environmental Pollution*. 233. 577-587.

7. FDA website, accessed on July 26, 2019. Available from www.fda.gov/cosmetics/cosmetic-ingredients/talc

8. Burns, Carla. 'Natural' or 'Organic' Cosmetics? Don't Trust Marketing Claims, Environmental Working Group. 2018. Accessed on July 27, 2019. Available from https://www.ewg.org/news-and-analysis/2018/01/natural-or-organic-cosmetics-don-t-trust-marketing-claims

9. Matta MK, Zusterzeel R, Pilli NR, et al. Effect of Sunscreen Application Under Maximal Use Conditions on Plasma Concentration of Sunscreen Active Ingredients: A Randomized Clinical Trial. JAMA. Published online May 06, 2019321(21):2082–2091.

10. Ruszkiewicz JA, Pinkas A, Ferrer B, Peres TV, Tsatsakis A, Aschner M. Neurotoxic effect of active ingredients in sunscreen products, a contemporary review. *Toxicol Rep.* 2017;4:245–259. Published 2017 May 27.

11. Baker JL, Edlund A. Exploiting the Oral Microbiome to Prevent Tooth Decay: Has Evolution Already Provided the Best Tools?. *Front Microbiol.* 2019;9:3323. Published 2019 Jan 11.

12. Kellesarian, S.V., Malignaggi, V.R., Kellesarian, T.V., Al-Kheraif, A.A., Alwageet, M.M., Malmstrom, H., Romanos, G.E., & Javed, F. (2017). Association between periodontal disease and polycystic ovary syndrome: a systematic review. International Journal of Impotence Research, 29, 89-95.

13. Nayak, P. A., Nayak, U. A., & Khandelwal, V. (2014). The effect of xylitol on dental caries and oral flora. *Clinical, cosmetic and investigational dentistry,* 6, 89-94.

14. Salminen, Seppo & Salminen, E & Koivistoinen, P & Bridges, J & Marks, Vincent. (1985). Gut microflora interactions with xylitol in the mouse, rat and man. *Food and chemical toxicology:* an international journal published for the British Industrial Biological Research Association. 23. 985-90.

15. Adams SE, Arnold D, Murphy B, et al. A randomised clinical study to determine the effect of a toothpaste containing enzymes and proteins on plaque oral microbiome ecology. *Sci Rep.* 2017;7:43344. Published 2017 Feb 27.

16. Chuang LC, Huang CS, Ou-Yang LW, Lin SY. Probiotic Lactobacillus paracasei effect on cariogenic bacterial flora. *Clin Oral Investig.* 2011;15(4):471–476.

17. Academy of General Dentistry. "Toothpaste with triclosan/copolymer kills harmful germs, study finds." *ScienceDaily,* 18 May 2010. Accessed on June 3, 2019 at www.sciencedaily.com/releases/2010/04/100413121334.htm

18. Alshehri FA. The use of mouthwash containing essential oils (LISTERINE®) to improve oral health: A systematic review. *Saudi Dent J.* 2018;30(1):2–6.

19. Kapil, V., Haydar, S. M., Pearl, V., Lundberg, J. O., Weitzberg, E., & Ahluwalia, A. (2013). Physiological role for nitrate-reducing oral bacteria in blood pressure control. *Free radical biology & medicine,* 55, 93-100.

20. Kaumudi J. Joshipura, Francisco J. Muñoz-Torres, Evangelia Morou-Bermudez, Rakesh P. Patel. Over-the-counter mouthwash use and risk of pre-diabetes/diabetes, *Nitric Oxide,* Volume 71, 2017, Pages 14-20.

21. Gareth Willis, Rosie Hocking, Maneesh Udiawar, Aled Rees, Philip James. Oxidative stress and nitric oxide in polycystic ovary syndrome, *Nitric Oxide,* Volume 27, Supplement, 2012, Page S28.

Chapter 12

1. Katrine Hass Rubin, Dorte Glintborg, Mads Nybo, Bo Abrahamsen, Marianne Andersen; Development and Risk Factors of Type 2 Diabetes in a Nationwide Population of Women With Polycystic Ovary Syndrome, *The Journal of Clinical Endocrinology & Metabolism,* Volume 102, Issue 10, 1 October 2017, Pages 3848–3857.

2. Umpleby, A.M., Shojaee-Moradie, F., Fielding, B.A., Li, X., Marino, A., Alsini, N., Isherwood, C.M., Jackson, N.C., Ahmad, A., Stolinski, M., Lovegrove, J.A., Johnsen, S., Mendis, A.S., Wright, J., Wilinska, M.E., Hovorka, R., Bell, J.D., Thomas, E.L., Frost, G.S., & Griffin, B.A. (2017). Impact of liver fat on the differential partitioning of hepatic triacylglycerol into VLDL subclasses on high and low sugar diets. *Clinical science,* 131 21, 2561-2573.

3. Knüppel, A., Shipley, M. J., Llewellyn, C. H., & Brunner, E. J. (2017). Sugar intake from sweet food and beverages, common mental disorder and depression: prospective findings from the Whitehall II study. *Scientific reports,* 7(1), 6287.

4. de la Monte, S. M., & Wands, J. R. (2008). Alzheimer's disease is type 3 diabetes-evidence reviewed. *Journal of diabetes science and technology,* 2(6), 1101-13.

5. Emilie Friberg, Alice Wallin and Alicja Wolk. Sucrose, High-Sugar Foods, and Risk of Endometrial Cancer—a Population-Based Cohort Study. *Cancer Epidemiology Biomarkers & Prevention.* September 1, 2011 (20) (9) 1831-1837.

6. Jiang, Y., Pan, Y., Rhea, P. R., Tan, L., Gagea, M., Cohen, L., Fischer, S. M., ... Yang, P. (2016). A Sucrose-Enriched Diet Promotes Tumorigenesis in Mammary Gland in Part through the 12-Lipoxygenase Pathway. *Cancer research,* 76(1), 24-9.

7. Guy E. Townsend, Weiwei Han, Nathan D. Schwalm, Varsha Raghavan, Natasha A. Barry, Andrew L. Goodman, Eduardo A. Groisman. Dietary sugar silences a colonization factor in a mammalian gut symbiont, *Proceedings of the National Academy of Sciences* Jan 2019, 116 (1) 233-238.

8. Chavarro JE, Rich-Edwards JW, Rosner BA, Willett WC. A prospective study of dietary carbohydrate quantity and quality in relation to risk of ovulatory infertility. *Eur J Clin Nutr.* 2009; 63(1):78–86.

9. Wiss DA, Avena N, Rada P. Sugar Addiction: From Evolution to Revolution. *Front Psychiatry.* 2018; 9:545. Published 2018 Nov 7.

10. Kwok CS, Boekholdt SM, Lentjes MAH, *et al.* Habitual chocolate consumption and risk of cardiovascular disease among healthy men and women, *Heart*, 2015; 101:1279-1287.

11. Saftlas AF, Triche EW, Beydoun H, Bracken MB. Does chocolate intake during pregnancy reduce the risks of preeclampsia and gestational hypertension?. *Ann Epidemiol*. 2010; 20(8):584–591.

12. Suez, Jotham & Korem, Tal & Zeevi, David & Zilberman-Schapira, Gili & A Thaiss, Christoph & Maza, Ori & Israeli, David & Zmora, Niv & Gilad, Shlomit & Weinberger, Adina & Kuperman, Yael & Harmelin, Alon & Kolodkin-Gal, Ilana & Shapiro, Hagit & Halpern, Zamir & Segal, Eran & Elinav, Eran. (2014). Artificial Sweeteners Induce Glucose Intolerance by Altering the Gut Microbiota. *Nature*. 70.

13. GBD 2016 Alcohol Collaborators. Alcohol use and burden for 195 countries and territories, 1990–2016: a systematic analysis for the Global Burden of Disease Study 2016. *The Lancet*. 23 Aug 2018.

14. Kumarendran, B., O'Reilly, M. W., Manolopoulos, K. N., Toulis, K. A., Gokhale, K. M., Sitch, A. J., Wijeyaratne, C. N., Coomarasamy, A., Arlt, W., ... Nirantharakumar, K. (2018). Polycystic ovary syndrome, androgen excess, and the risk of nonalcoholic fatty liver disease in women: A longitudinal study based on a United Kingdom primary care database. *PLoS medicine*, 15(3), e1002542.

15. Petta S, Ciresi A, Bianco J, Geraci V, Boemi R, Galvano L, et al. Insulin resistance and hyperandrogenism drive steatosis and fibrosis risk in young females with PCOS. *PLoS One*. 2017;12(11): e0186136

16. Taisto Sarkola, Tatsushige Fukunaga, Heikki Mäkisalo, C. J. Peter Eriksson, Acute effect of alcohol on androgens in premenopausal women, *Alcohol and Alcoholism*, Volume 35, Issue 1, January 2000, Pages 84–90.

17. Engen PA, Green SJ, Voigt RM, Forsyth CB, Keshavarzian A. The Gastrointestinal Microbiome: Alcohol Effects on the Composition of Intestinal Microbiota. *Alcohol Res*. 2015;37(2):223–236.

18. Bishehsari F, Magno E, Swanson G, et al. Alcohol and Gut-Derived Inflammation. *Alcohol Res*. 2017;38(2):163–171.

19. Grant BF, Chou SP, Saha TD, et al. Prevalence of 12-Month Alcohol Use, High-Risk Drinking, and DSM-IV Alcohol Use Disorder in the United States, 2001-2002 to 2012-2013: Results From the National Epidemiologic Survey on Alcohol and Related Conditions. *JAMA Psychiatry*. 2017; 74(9):911–923.

20. Bahar Azemati, Sujatha Rajaram, Karen Jaceldo-Siegl, Joan Sabate, David Shavlik, Gary E Fraser, Ella H Haddad, Animal-Protein Intake Is Associated with Insulin Resistance in Adventist Health Study 2 (AHS-2) Calibration Substudy Participants: A Cross-Sectional Analysis, *Current Developments in Nutrition*, Volume 1, Issue 4, April 2017, e000299.

21. Chavarro, Jorge E. et al. Protein intake and ovulatory infertility, *American Journal of Obstetrics & Gynecology*, Volume 198, Issue 2, 210.e1 - 210.e7.

22. Murphy, E. A., Velazquez, K. T., & Herbert, K. M. (2015). Influence of high-fat diet on gut microbiota: a driving force for chronic disease risk. *Current opinion in clinical nutrition and metabolic care*, 18(5), 515-20.

23. Teng, K. T., Chang, C. Y., Chang, L. F., & Nesaretnam, K. (2014). Modulation of obesity-induced inflammation by dietary fats: mechanisms and clinical evidence. *Nutrition journal*, 13, 12.

24. Turnbaugh, P.J., Ley, R.E., Mahowald, M.A., Magrini, V., Mardis, E.R., & Gordon, J.I. (2006). An obesity-associated gut microbiome with increased capacity for energy harvest. *Nature*, 444, 1027-1031.

25. Zhang, C., Zhang, M., Pang, X., Zhao, Y., Wang, L., & Zhao, L. (2012). Structural resilience of the gut microbiota in adult mice under high-fat dietary perturbations. *The ISME Journal*, 6, 1848-1857.

26. Murphy, E. A., Velazquez, K. T., & Herbert, K. M. (2015). Influence of high-fat diet on gut microbiota: a driving force for chronic disease risk. *Current opinion in clinical nutrition and metabolic care*, 18(5), 515-20.

27. Daley CA, Abbott A, Doyle PS, Nader GA, Larson S. A review of fatty acid profiles and antioxidant content in grass-fed and grain-fed beef. *Nutr J*. 2010;9:10. Published 2010 Mar 10.

28. Minger, Denise. 4 Hidden Dangers of Pork, Healthline. June 22, 2017. Accessed June 6, 2019 at https://www.healthline.com/nutrition/is-pork-bad

29. Audrey J Gaskins, Rajeshwari Sundaram, Germaine M Buck Louis, Jorge E Chavarro, Seafood Intake, Sexual Activity, and Time to Pregnancy, *The Journal of Clinical Endocrinology & Metabolism*, Volume 103, Issue 7, July 2018, Pages 2680–2688.

30. Pourafshar, Shirin & S. Akhavan, Neda & S. George, Kelli & Foley, Elizabeth & Johnson, Sarah & Keshavarz, Behnam & Navaei, Negin & Davoudi, Anis & A. Clark, Elizabeth & Arjmandi, Bahram. (2018). Egg consumption may improve factors associated with glycemic control and insulin sensitivity in adults with pre- and type II diabetes. *Food & Function*. 9.

31. Marie A. Caudill, Barbara J. Strupp, Laura Muscalu, Julie E. H. Nevins, Richard L. Canfield. Maternal choline supplementation during the third trimester of pregnancy improves infant information processing speed: a randomized, double-blind, controlled feeding study. *The FASEB Journal*, 2017; fj.201700692RR.

32. Qin C, Lv J, Guo Y on behalf of the China Kadoorie Biobank Collaborative Group, et al. Associations of egg consumption with cardiovascular disease in a cohort study of 0.5 million Chinese adults, *Heart* 2018;104:1756-1763.

33. J.E. Chavarro, J.W. Rich-Edwards, B. Rosner, W.C. Willett, A prospective study of dairy foods intake and anovulatory infertility, *Human Reproduction*, Volume 22, Issue 5, May 2007, Pages 1340–1347.

34. Rajaeieh, G., Marasi, M., Shahshahan, Z., Hassanbeigi, F., & Safavi, S. M. (2014). The Relationship between Intake of Dairy Products and Polycystic Ovary Syndrome in Women Who Referred to Isfahan University of Medical Science Clinics in 2013. *International journal of preventive medicine*, 5(6), 687-94.

35. Adebamowo CA, Spiegelman D, Danby FW, et al. High school dietary dairy intake and teenage acne. *J Am Acad Dermatol.* 2005; 52:207-214.

36. (2011). Acne: Diet and acnegenesis. *Indian dermatology online journal*, 2(1), 2-5.

Chapter 13

1. Martin CK, Rosenbaum D, Han H, et al. Change in food cravings, food preferences, and appetite during a low-carbohydrate and low-fat diet. *Obesity (Silver Spring)*. 2011;19(10):1963-1970.

2. De Silva A, Salem V, Matthews PM, Dhillo WS. The use of functional MRI to study appetite control in the CNS. *Exp Diabetes Res.* 2012; 2012:764017.

3. Pelchat, M.L., Johnson, A.B., Chan, R.C., Valdez, J.N., & Ragland, J.D. (2004). Images of desire: food-craving activation during fMRI. *NeuroImage*, 23, 1486-1493.

4. Chao A, Grilo CM, White MA, Sinha R. Food cravings, food intake, and weight status in a community-based sample. *Eat Behav.* 2014;15(3):478-482.

5. Alcock, Joe & Maley, Carlo & Aktipis, C. (2014). Is eating behavior manipulated by the gastrointestinal microbiota? Evolutionary pressures and potential mechanisms. *BioEssays.* 36.

6. Hetherington, M.M., & Boyland, E. (2006). Short-term effects of chewing gum on snack intake and appetite. *Appetite*, 48, 397-401.

7. Vatansever-Ozen S, Tiryaki-Sonmez G, Bugdayci G, Ozen G. The effects of exercise on food intake and hunger: relationship with acylated ghrelin and leptin. *J Sports Sci Med.* 2011;10(2):283-291. Published 2011 Jun 1.

8. Hondorp, Shawn & Kleinman, Brighid & Hood, Megan & M. Nackers, Lisa & Corsica, Joyce. (2014). Mindfulness meditation as an intervention for binge eating, emotional eating, and weight loss: A systematic review. *Eating Behaviors.* 15.

9. S Westerterp-Plantenga, M & P G M Lejeune, M & Nijs, Ilse & van Ooijen, M & Kovacs, Eva. (2004). High protein intake sustains weight maintenance after weight loss in humans. International journal of obesity and related metabolic disorders: *Journal of the International Association for the Study of Obesity.* 28. 57-64.

10. Zheng J, Zheng S, Feng Q, Zhang Q, Xiao X. Dietary capsaicin and its anti-obesity potency: from mechanism to clinical implications. *Biosci Rep.* 2017; 37(3):BSR20170286. Published 2017 May 11.

11. Nguyen V, Cooper L, Lowndes J, et al. Popcorn is more satiating than potato chips in normal-weight adults. *Nutr J.* 2012;11:71. Published 2012 Sep 14.

12. Hyun-seok Kim, MD, MPH; Kalpesh G. Patel, MD; Evan Orosz, DO; et al. Time Trends in the Prevalence of Celiac Disease and Gluten-Free Diet in the US Population: Results From the National Health and Nutrition Examination Surveys 2009-2014. *JAMA Intern Med.* 2016;176(11):1716-1717.

13. Shah S, Leffler D. Celiac disease: an underappreciated issue in women's health. *Womens Health (Lond).* 2010;6(5):753-766.

14. Admou, B., Essaadouni, L., Krati, K., Zaher, K., Sbihi, M., Chabaa, L., Belaabidia, B., ... Alaoui-Yazidi, A. (2012). Atypical celiac disease: from recognizing to managing. *Gastroenterology research and practice*, 2012, 637187.

15. Singh, Prashant & Arora, Shubhangi & Lal, Suman & Strand, Tor & Makharia, Govind. (2015). Celiac Disease in Women With Infertility: A Meta-Analysis. *Journal of Clinical Gastroenterology.*

16. Lyngsø J, Ramlau-Hansen CH, Bay B, Ingerslev HJ, Hulman A, Kesmodel US. Association between coffee or caffeine consumption and fecundity and fertility: a systematic review and dose-response meta-analysis. *Clin Epidemiol.* 2017;9:699-719. Published 2017 Dec 15.

17. Centers for Disease Control and Prevention. Tobacco-Related Mortality. Article accessed on June 8, 2019. Available from https://www.cdc.gov/tobacco/data_statistics/fact_sheets/health_effects/tobacco_related_mortality/index.htm

18. Shah T, Sullivan K, Carter J. Sudden infant death syndrome and reported maternal smoking during pregnancy. *Am J Public Health.* 2006;96(10):1757-1759.

19. Kapaya M, D'Angelo DV, Tong VT, et al. Use of Electronic Vapor Products Before, During, and After Pregnancy Among Women with a Recent Live Birth — Oklahoma and Texas, 2015. *MMWR Morb Mortal Wkly Rep,* 2019; 68:189-194.

20. R Whittington, Julie & M Simmons, Pamela & M Phillips, Amy & K Gammill, Sarah & Cen, Ruiqi & Magann, Everett & M Cardenas, Victor. (2018). The Use of Electronic Cigarettes in Pregnancy: A Review of the Literature. *Obstetrical & gynecological survey.* 73. 544-549.

21. Wickström R. Effects of nicotine during pregnancy: human and experimental evidence. *Curr Neuropharmacol.* 2007; 5(3):213-222.

22. Kennedy AE, Kandalam S, Olivares-Navarrete R, Dickinson AJG. E-cigarette aerosol exposure can cause craniofacial defects in Xenopus laevis embryos and mammalian neural crest cells. *PLoS One.* 2017;12(9):e0185729. Published 2017 Sep 28.

23. Prud'homme M, Cata R, Jutras-Aswad D. Cannabidiol as an Intervention for Addictive Behaviors: A Systematic Review of the Evidence. *Subst Abuse.* 2015; 9:33–38. Published 2015 May 21.
24. National Environmental Health Association, Third Hand Smoke. Accessed on June 8, 2019. Available from https://www.neha.org/eh-topics/air-quality-0/third-hand-smoke.
25. Rehan VK, Sakurai R, Torday JS. Thirdhand smoke: a new dimension to the effects of cigarette smoke on the developing lung. *Am J Physiol Lung Cell Mol Physiol.* 2011;301(1):L1–L8.
26. Maciej L. Goniewicz, Lily Lee, Electronic Cigarettes Are a Source of Thirdhand Exposure to Nicotine, *Nicotine & Tobacco Research*, Volume 17, Issue 2, February 2015, Pages 256–258.
27. Battista, N., Meccariello, R., Cobellis, G., Fasano, S., Tommaso, M.D., Pirazzi, V., Konje, J.C., Pierantoni, R., & Maccarrone, M. (2012). The role of endocannabinoids in gonadal function and fertility along the evolutionary axis. *Molecular and Cellular Endocrinology*, 355, 1-14.
28. Habayeb, O.M., Taylor, A.H., Evans, M.D., Cooke, M.S., Taylor, D.J., Bell, S.C., & Konje, J.C. (2004). Plasma levels of the endocannabinoid anandamide in women--a potential role in pregnancy maintenance and labor? *The Journal of clinical endocrinology and metabolism*, 89 11, 5482-7 .
29. Friedrich J, Khatib D, Parsa K, Santopietro A, Gallicano GI. The grass isn't always greener: The effects of cannabis on embryological development. *BMC Pharmacol Toxicol.* 2016; 17(1):45. Published 2016 Sep 29.
30. Metz TD, Allshouse AA, Hogue CJ, et al. Maternal marijuana use, adverse pregnancy outcomes, and neonatal morbidity. *Am J Obstet Gynecol.* 2017; 217(4):478.e1–478.e8.
31. Leemaqz, S.Y., Dekker, G., McCowan, L.M., Kenny, L.C., Myers, J.E., Simpson, N., Cutfield, W.S., & Roberts, C.T. (2016). Maternal marijuana use has independent effects on risk for spontaneous preterm birth but not other common late pregnancy complications. *Reproductive toxicology*, 62, 77-86 .
32. Barros, M.C., Guinsburg, R., Peres, C.D., Mitsuhiro, S.S., Chalem, E., & Laranjeira, R. (2006). Exposure to marijuana during pregnancy alters neurobehavior in the early neonatal period. *The Journal of pediatrics*, 149 6, 781-7.
33. Burkman, Lani & L. Bodziak, M & Schuel, Herbert & Palaszewski, Dawn & Gurunatha, R. (2003). Marijuana (MJ) impacts sperm function both in vivo and in vitro: semen analyses from men smoking marijuana. *Fertility and Sterility*. 80. 231-231.

Chapter 14

1. Ormesher, L., Myers, J.E., Chmiel, C., Wareing, M., Greenwood, S.L., Tropea, T., Lundberg, J.O., Weitzberg, E., Nihlén, C., Sibley, C.P., Johnstone, E.D., & Cottrell, E. (2018). Effects of dietary nitrate supplementation, from beetroot juice, on blood pressure in hypertensive pregnant women: A randomised, double-blind, placebo-controlled feasibility trial. *Nitric oxide: biology and chemistry*, 80, 37-44 .
2. Cottrell, Elizabeth & Garrod, Ainslie & Wareing, Mark & Dilworth, Mark & Finn-Sell, Sarah & Greenwood, Susan & Baker, Philip & Sibley, Colin. (2014). Supplementation with inorganic nitrate during pregnancy improves maternal uterine artery function and placental efficiency in mice. *Placenta*. 35. A21.
3. Marco, M.L., Heeney, D.D., Binda, S., Cifelli, C.J., Cotter, P.D., Foligné, B., Gänzle, M.G., Kort, R., Pasin, G., Pihlanto, A., Smid, E.J., & Hutkins, R.W. (2017). Health benefits of fermented foods: microbiota and beyond. *Current opinion in biotechnology*, 44, 94-102.
4. Karamali, M., Eghbalpour, S., Rajabi, S., Jamilian, M., Bahmani, F., Tajabadi-Ebrahimi, M., Keneshlou, F., Mirhashemi, SM., Chamani, M., Hashem Gelougerdi, S., Asemi, Z. (2018). Effects of Probiotic Supplementation on Hormonal Profiles, Biomarkers of Inflammation and Oxidative Stress in Women With Polycystic Ovary Syndrome: A Randomized, Double-Blind, Placebo-Controlled Trial. *Arch Iran Med.* 2018 Jan 1; 21(1):1-7.
5. Edwards SM, Cunningham SA, Dunlop AL, Corwin EJ. The Maternal Gut Microbiome During Pregnancy. *MCN Am J Matern Child Nurs.* 2017; 42(6):310–317.
6. Jorge E. Chavarro, Lidia Mínguez-Alarcón, Yu-Han Chiu, Audrey J. Gaskins, Irene Souter, Paige L. Williams, Antonia M. Calafat, Russ Hauser. Soy Intake Modifies the Relation Between Urinary Bisphenol A Concentrations and Pregnancy Outcomes Among Women Undergoing Assisted Reproduction. *The Journal of Clinical Endocrinology & Metabolism*, 2016; jc.2015-3473.
7. Grant, P. (2010), Spearmint herbal tea has significant anti-androgen effects in polycystic ovarian syndrome. a randomized controlled trial. *Phytother. Res.*, 24: 186-188.
8. Akdoğan, M.V., Tamer, M.N., Cüre, E., Cüre, M.C., Köroğlu, B.K., & Delibaş, N. (2007). Effect of spearmint (Mentha spicata Labiatae) teas on androgen levels in women with hirsutism. *Phytotherapy research: PTR*, 21 5, 444-7.
9. Terman, M. and Terman, J.S., Controlled Trial of Naturalistic Dawn Simulation and Negative Air Ionization for Seasonal Affective Disorder. *American Journal of Psychiatry* (2006) 163:12, 2126-2133.
10. Danilenko, Konstantin & Ivanova, I.A.. (2015). Dawn simulation vs. bright light in seasonal affective disorder: Treatment effects and subjective preference. *Journal of affective disorders*. 180. 87-89.

11. Leppamaki S, Meesters Y, Haukka J, et al. Effect of simulated dawn on quality of sleep—a community-based trial. *BMC Psychiatry.* 2003; 3:14.

12. Thorn, L. et al. The effect of dawn simulation on the cortisol response to awakening in healthy participants. *Psychoneuroendocrinology,* Volume 29 , Issue 7, 925 - 930.

13. Shin-Jung Park & Hiromi Tokura (1999) Bright Light Exposure During the Daytime Affects Circadian Rhythms of Urinary Melatonin and Salivary Immunoglobulin A, *Chronobiology International,* 16:3,359-371.

14. Nair, R., & Maseeh, A. (2012). Vitamin D: The "sunshine" vitamin. *Journal of pharmacology & pharmacotherapeutics,* 3(2), 118-26.

15. University of Southampton. (2014, January 17). Here comes the sun to lower your blood pressure. *ScienceDaily.* Retrieved November 7, 2018 from www.sciencedaily.com/releases/2014/01/140117090139.htm

16. Matsui, M. S., Pelle, E., Dong, K., & Pernodet, N. (2016). Biological Rhythms in the Skin. International journal of molecular sciences, 17(6), 801.

17. Krishna, Meera & Joseph, Annu & Litto Thomas, Philip & Dsilva, Belinda & M Pillai, Sathy & Laloraya, Malini. (2017). Impaired Arginine Metabolism Coupled to a Defective Redox Conduit Contributes to Low Plasma Nitric Oxide in Polycystic Ovary Syndrome. *Cellular physiology and biochemistry: international journal of experimental cellular physiology, biochemistry, and pharmacology.* 43. 1880-1892.

18. Smith Conway, Karen & Trudeau, Jennifer. (2018). Sunshine, Fertility and Racial Disparities. SSRN *Electronic Journal.*

19. Lin MW, Wu MH. The role of vitamin D in polycystic ovary syndrome. *Indian J Med Res.* 2015; 142(3):238–240.

20. Plataforma SINC. (2017, March 8). How much sun is good for our health? *ScienceDaily.* Retrieved November 7, 2018 from www.sciencedaily.com/releases/2017/03/170308083938.htm

21. Maria-Antonia Serrano, Javier Cañada, Juan Carlos Moreno, Gonzalo Gurrea. Solar ultraviolet doses and vitamin D in a northern mid-latitude. *Science of The Total Environment,* 2017; 574: 744.

22. Hartman, S. J., Nelson, S. H., & Weiner, L. S. (2018). Patterns of Fitbit Use and Activity Levels Throughout a Physical Activity Intervention: Exploratory Analysis from a Randomized Controlled Trial. *JMIR mHealth and uHealth,* 6(2), e29.

23. Gareth Willis, Rosie Hocking, Maneesh Udiawar, Aled Rees, Philip James. Oxidative stress and nitric oxide in polycystic ovary syndrome, *Nitric Oxide,* Volume 27, Supplement, 2012, Page S28.

24. Beata Banaszewska, Joanna Wrotyńska-Barczyńska, Robert Z. Spaczynski, Leszek Pawelczyk, Antoni J. Duleba. Effects of Resveratrol on Polycystic Ovary Syndrome: A Double-blind, Randomized, Placebo-controlled Trial. *The Journal of Clinical Endocrinology & Metabolism,* 2016; jc.2016-1858.

25. Mukhri Hamdan, Keith T. Jones, Ying Cheong, Simon I. R. Lane. The sensitivity of the DNA damage checkpoint prevents oocyte maturation in endometriosis. *Scientific Reports,* 2016; 6: 36994.

26. Zhang, Ying & Liu, Jin & Chen, Xiaoqiang & Chen, Oliver. (2018). Ubiquinol is superior to ubiquinone to enhance Coenzyme Q10 status in older men. *Food & Function.* 9.

27. Özcan P, Fıçıcıoğlu C, Kizilkale O, et al. Can Coenzyme Q10 supplementation protect the ovarian reserve against oxidative damage?. *J Assist Reprod Genet.* 2016;33(9):1223–1230.

28. Xu Y, Nisenblat V, Lu C, et al. Pretreatment with coenzyme Q10 improves ovarian response and embryo quality in low-prognosis young women with decreased ovarian reserve: a randomized controlled trial. *Reprod Biol Endocrinol.* 2018;16(1):29. Published 2018 Mar 27.

29. Ben-Meir A, Burstein E, Borrego-Alvarez A, et al. Coenzyme Q10 restores oocyte mitochondrial function and fertility during reproductive aging. *Aging Cell.* 2015;14(5):887–895.

Chapter 15

1. Steinemann, Anne. (2016). Fragranced consumer products: exposures and effects from emissions. *Air Quality, Atmosphere & Health.* 9.

2. Carignan, C.C., Mínguez-Alarcón, L., Butt, C.M., Williams, P.L., Meeker, J.D., Stapleton, H.M., Toth, T., Ford, J.B., & Hauser, R. (2017). Urinary Concentrations of Organophosphate Flame Retardant Metabolites and Pregnancy Outcomes among Women Undergoing in Vitro Fertilization. *Environmental health perspectives.*

3. Sherriff A, Farrow A, Golding J, Henderson J. Frequent use of chemical household products is associated with persistent wheezing in pre-school age children. *Thorax.* 2005; 60(1):45–49.

4. Singla, Veena. (2016, September 13) Toxic Dust: The Dangerous Chemical Brew in Every Home. *National Resource Defense Council.* Available from: https://www.nrdc.org/experts/veena-singla/toxic-dust-dangerous-chemical-brew-every-home

5. Layton et al. Migration of Contaminated Soil and Airborne Particulates to Indoor Dust. *Environmental Science & Technology,* 2009; 090924111235017.

6. Environmental Protection Agency, Indoor Air Quality (IAQ). Accessed on June 13, 2019. Available from https://www.epa.gov/indoor-air-quality-iaq.

7. Vijayan, V. K., Paramesh, H., Salvi, S. S., & Dalal, A. A. (2015). Enhancing indoor air quality -The air filter advantage. *Lung India : official organ of Indian Chest Society*, 32(5), 473-9.
8. Carré, J., Gatimel, N., Moreau, J., Parinaud, J., & Léandri, R.D. (2017). Does air pollution play a role in infertility?: a systematic review. *Environmental health : a global access science source*.
9. Singer, Brett & Zarin Pass, Rebecca & W. Delp, William & Lorenzetti, David & L. Maddalena, Randy. (2017). Pollutant concentrations and emission rates from natural gas cooking burners without and with range hood exhaust in nine California homes. *Building and Environment*. 122.
10. Langlois PH, Lee M, Lupo PJ, Rahbar MH, Cortez RK. Residential radon and birth defects: A population-based assessment. *Birth Defects Res A Clin Mol Teratol*. 2016; 106(1):5-15.
11. Bassil, K. L., Vakil, C., Sanborn, M., Cole, D. C., Kaur, J. S., & Kerr, K. J. (2007). Cancer health effects of pesticides: systematic review. *Canadian family physician Medecin de famille canadien*, 53(10), 1704-11.
12. Marcia G. Nishioka,*, Hazel M. Burkholder, and, Marielle C. Brinkman, and Robert G. Lewis. Distribution of 2,4-Dichlorophenoxyacetic Acid in Floor Dust throughout Homes Following Homeowner and Commercial Lawn Applications: Quantitative Effects of Children, Pets, and Shoes. *Environmental Science & Technology*. 1999 33 (9), 1359-1365.

Chapter 16

1. Annan JJ, Gudi A, Bhide P, Shah A, Homburg R. Biochemical pregnancy during assisted conception: a little bit pregnant. . 2013;5(4):269–274.
2. Optimizing natural fertility: a committee opinion. *Fertility and Sterility*, Volume 100, Issue 3, 631 - 637.
3. King R, Dempsey M, Valentine KA. Measuring sperm backflow following female orgasm: a new method. . 2016; 6:31927. Published 2016 Oct 25.
4. Tummon, Ian & Gavrilova-Jordan, Larisa & C Allemand, Michael & Session, Donna. (2005). Polycystic ovaries and ovarian hyperstimulation syndrome: A systematic review. *Acta obstetricia et gynecologica Scandinavica*. 84. 611-6.
5. Hu, Shifu & Yu, Qiong & Wang, Yingying & Wang, Mei & Xia, Wei & Zhu, Changhong. (2018). Letrozole versus clomiphene citrate in polycystic ovary syndrome: a meta-analysis of randomized controlled trials. *Archives of Gynecology and Obstetrics*. 297.
6. Hashim, H.A. (2017). Management of Women with Clomifene Citrate Resistant Polycystic Ovary Syndrome – An Evidence Based Approach.
7. Legro, Richard & G Brzyski, Robert & Diamond, Michael & Coutifaris, Christos & Schlaff, William & Casson, Peter & M Christman, Gregory & Huang, Hao & Yan, Qingshang & Alvero, Ruben & Haisenleder, Daniel & T Barnhart, Kurt & Bates, Gordon & Usadi, Rebecca & Lucidi, Scott & Baker, Valerie & Trussell, J.C. & A Krawetz, Stephen & Snyder, Peter & Zhang, Heping. (2014). Letrozole Versus Clomiphene for Infertility in the Polycystic Ovary Syndrome. *The New England journal of medicine*. 371. 119-129.
8. Hajishafiha M, Dehghan M, Kiarang N, Sadegh-Asadi N, Shayegh SN, Ghasemi-Rad M. Combined letrozole and clomiphene versus letrozole and clomiphene alone in infertile patients with polycystic ovary syndrome [published correction appears in Drug Des Devel Ther. 2017 Apr 28;11:1367]. . 2013; 7:1427-1431. Published 2013 Dec 3.
9. (2014). Metformin use in women with polycystic ovary syndrome. , (6), 56.
10. Liv Guro Engen Hanem, Solhild Stridsklev, Pétur B Júlíusson, Øyvind Salvesen, Mathieu Roelants, Sven M Carlsen, Rønnaug Ødegård, Eszter Vanky; Metformin Use in PCOS Pregnancies Increases the Risk of Offspring Overweight at 4 Years of Age: Follow-Up of Two RCTs, *The Journal of Clinical Endocrinology & Metabolism*, Volume 103, Issue 4, 1 April 2018, Pages 1612–1621.
11. Rasmussen, C. B., & Lindenberg, S. (2014). The effect of liraglutide on weight loss in women with polycystic ovary syndrome: an observational study. , , 140.
12. Loy SL, Chan JK, Wee PH, et al. Maternal Circadian Eating Time and Frequency Are Associated with Blood Glucose Concentrations during Pregnancy. . 2017;147(1):70–77.
13. Marie A. Caudill, Barbara J. Strupp, Laura Muscalu, Julie E. H. Nevins, Richard L. Canfield. Maternal choline supplementation during the third trimester of pregnancy improves infant information processing speed: a randomized, double-blind, controlled feeding study. *The FASEB Journal*, 2017; fj.201700692RR.
14. Zarean E, Tarjan A. Effect of Magnesium Supplement on Pregnancy Outcomes: A Randomized Control Trial. . 2017;6:109. Published 2017 Aug 31.
15. Feig, Denice & E Donovan, Lois & Corcoy, Rosa & Murphy, Kellie & Amiel, Stephanie & F Hunt, Katharine & Asztalos, Elisabeth & Barrett, Jon & Sanchez, Johanna & De Leiva, Alberto & Hod, Moshe & Jovanovic, Lois & Keely, Erin & McManus, Ruth & Hutton, Eileen & Meek, Claire & A Stewart, Zoe & Wysocki, Tim & O'Brien, Robert & Pragnell, Marlon. (2017). Continuous glucose monitoring in pregnant women with type 1 diabetes (CONCEPTT): A multicentre international randomised controlled trial. *The Lancet*. 390.

16. Chakraborty, P., Goswami, S. K., Rajani, S., Sharma, S., Kabir, S. N., Chakravarty, B., & Jana, K. (2013). Recurrent pregnancy loss in polycystic ovary syndrome: role of hyperhomocysteinemia and insulin resistance. , (5), e64446.

17. Kamalanathan S, Sahoo JP, Sathyapalan T. Pregnancy in polycystic ovary syndrome. . 2013;17(1):37–43.

18. Kaur R, Gupta K. Endocrine dysfunction and recurrent spontaneous abortion: An overview. . 2016;6(2):79–83.

19. Krieg, Sacha A. et al. Environmental exposure to endocrine-disrupting chemicals and miscarriage, *Fertility and Sterility*, (2016) Volume 106, Issue 4, 941 - 947.

20. Hussain M, El-Hakim S, Cahill DJ. Progesterone supplementation in women with otherwise unexplained recurrent miscarriages. . 2012;5(3):248–251.

21. Kolte AM, Olsen LR, Mikkelsen EM, Christiansen OB, Nielsen HS. Depression and emotional stress is highly prevalent among women with recurrent pregnancy loss. . 2015;30(4):777–782.

Bonus Section on Male Fertility

1. Palmer NO, Bakos HW, Fullston T, Lane M. Impact of obesity on male fertility, sperm function and molecular composition. *Spermatogenesis*. 2012;2(4):253–263.

2. Albert Salas-Huetos, Rocío Moraleda, Simona Giardina, Ester Anton, Joan Blanco, Jordi Salas-Salvadó, Mònica Bulló, Effect of nut consumption on semen quality and functionality in healthy men consuming a Western-style diet: a randomized controlled trial, *The American Journal of Clinical Nutrition*, Volume 108, Issue 5, November 2018, Pages 953–962.

3. Safarinejad MR, Safarinejad S. The roles of omega-3 and omega-6 fatty acids in idiopathic male infertility. *Asian J Androl*. 2012;14(4):514–515.

4. Wang L, Yang Y, Liu F, *et al*. Paternal smoking and spontaneous abortion: a population-based retrospective cohort study among non-smoking women aged 20–49 years in rural China J *Epidemiol Community Health* 2018;72:783-789.

5. Ji, B.T., Shu, X., Linet, M.S., Zheng, W., Wacholder, S., Gao, Y., Ying, D., & Jin, F. (1997). Paternal cigarette smoking and the risk of childhood cancer among offspring of nonsmoking mothers. *Journal of the National Cancer Institute*, 89 3, 238-44 .

6. Lijuan Zhao, Lizhang Chen, Tubao Yang, Lesan Wang, Tingting Wang, Senmao Zhang, Letao Chen, Ziwei Ye, Zan Zheng, Jiabi Qin. Parental smoking and the risk of congenital heart defects in offspring: An updated meta-analysis of observational studies. *European Journal of Preventive Cardiology*, 2019.

7. Tremellen K. Oxidative stress and male infertility--a clinical perspective. *Hum Reprod Update*. 2008 May-Jun;14(3):243-58.

8. Haghighian, Hossein Khadem et al. Randomized, triple-blind, placebo-controlled clinical trial examining the effects of alpha-lipoic acid supplement on the spermatogram and seminal oxidative stress in infertile men, *Fertility and Sterility*, Volume 104, Issue 2, 318 - 324.

9. Tremellen K. Gut Endotoxin Leading to a Decline IN Gonadal function (GELDING)- a novel theory for the development of late onset hypogonadism in obese men. *Basic Clin Androl*. 2016 Jun 22;26:7.

10. Tremellen, Kelton & McPhee, Natalie & Pearce, Karma & Bedson, Sven & Schedlowski, Manfred & Engler, Harald. (2017). Endotoxin initiated inflammation reduces testosterone production in men of reproductive age. *American Journal of Physiology - Endocrinology And Metabolism*. 314. ajpendo.00279.2017.

11. Maretti C, Cavallini G. The association of a probiotic with a prebiotic (Flortec, Bracco) to improve the quality/quantity of spermatozoa in infertile patients with idiopathic oligoasthenoteratospermia: a pilot study. *Andrology*. 2017 May; 5(3):439-444.

12. Valcarce, D.G., Genovés, S., Riesco, M.F., Martorell, P.M., Herráez, M.P., Ramon, D.M., & Robles, V. (2017). Probiotic administration improves sperm quality in asthenozoospermic human donors. *Beneficial microbes*, 8 2, 193-206 .

13. Dardmeh F, Alipour H, Gazerani P, van der Horst G, Brandsborg E, Nielsen HI. Lactobacillus rhamnosus PB01 (DSM 14870) supplementation affects markers of sperm kinematic parameters in a diet-induced obesity mice model. *PLoS One*. 2017;12(10):e0185964. Published 2017 Oct 10.

14. Cherry N, Moore H, McNamee R, *et al*. Occupation and male infertility: glycol ethers and other exposures, *Occupational and Environmental Medicine* 2008;**65**:708-714.

15. Yatsenko AN, Turek PJ. Reproductive genetics and the aging male. J Assist Reprod Genet. 2018 Jun;35(6):933-941.

Workbooks

1. Nobles, Carrie & Mendola, Pauline & Mumford, Sunni & I. Naimi, Ashley & H. Yeung, Edwina & Kim, Keewan & Park, Hyojun & Wilcox, Brian & M. Silver, Robert & Perkins, Neil & Sjaarda, Lindsey & Schisterman, Enrique. (2018). Preconception Blood Pressure Levels and Reproductive Outcomes in a Prospective Cohort of Women Attempting Pregnancy. *Hypertension*. 71.

2. Merviel P, Cabry R, Lourdel E, et al. Comparison of two preventive treatments for patients with recurrent miscarriages carrying a C677T methylenetetrahydrofolate reductase mutation: 5-year experience. *J Int Med Res*. 2017; 45(6):1720–1730.

3. Reading the new blood pressure guidelines. [Accessed November 6, 2018]; *Harvard's Men's Health Watch*. Available from: https://www.health.harvard.edu/heart-health/reading-the-new-blood-pressure-guidelines

Index

Acknowledgments

*E*very book is a team effort, and I am fortunate beyond measure to have an incredible tribe of people supporting me every step of the way.

To Julia Pastore, my eloquent editor, thank you for making sure that my words say what I want them to say.

Alison Voetsch, you connect people. Thank you for helping me get my voice out there to share critical information about PCOS and women's health with the wider world.

I would like the thank Joy Devins, Kyle Bliffert, Paul Larkin, Kelly Heim, Joseph Lehrberg, and the entire team at Pure Encapsulations for your ongoing support and especially for putting my books into the hands of as many women as possible. David Zava and Kate Placzek, your enthusiasm for my work means so much to me. And a huge thank you to the amazing teams at Quest Diagnostics, Cleveland HeartLab, ZRT Lab, and L-Nutra for always encouraging me and supporting my efforts to educate women about their hormonal health.

To the amazing network of women who are advocating for PCOS awareness, research, and education, thank you for all of your work. I am in awe of your passion and dedication, and I am honored to be a part of this movement. Let's continue doing great things together! To Sasha Ottey and the team at PCOS Challenge, you are an incredible organization of powerful women advocating for more research and recognition for this common but underfunded condition. To Megan Stewart and all the tireless advocates at PCOS Awareness, the work you do educating women about this widespread disorder and the attention you demand from lawmakers, researchers, and the medical community is invaluable. Amy Medling of PCOS Diva, you are a voice of hope for so many women with PCOS. Thank you for helping to get the word out about kinder, more natural, healthier, and more effective treatments. See you all at the next PCOS event!

There is an incredible community of doctors and researchers working to better understand PCOS. Kelton Tremellen, I am inspired by your research. Thank you for all of the time and energy that you and your research team have dedicated to proving the impacts that lifestyle and diet have on fertility. And, of course, thank you so much for contributing your knowledge of male fertility to this book. Sara Gottfried, I love sharing ideas and sharing the stage with you. Thank you for cheering me on as I delve deeper into this world of publishing. Lyn Patrick, thank you for building a community of environmental medical practitioners. I look forward to your conference every year!

To JJ Virgin and the entire MindShare community, you are my inspiration and source of perpetual encouragement. Thank you for showing me what is possible and challenging me to think bigger.

To the amazing staff of people who spend time every day at Integrative Medical Group of Irvine helping patients and keeping the lights on, you are the backbone of everything I do. At the end of the day, it's all about the patients, the people who trust us with their health. Thank you for the incredible kindness and service that you give. And to all of my patients, thank you for choosing me as your doctor. Caring for patients has been my life's work. I've been doing this longer than I sometimes care to admit, but it never gets old or boring. Every day, I feel renewed by the deep responsibility and honor that comes with helping you on your ongoing journeys to wellness.

And of course, last but never least, I need to send a huge thank you to all of my dearest friends and family. Functional Medicine Babes, thanks for your bottomless love and warm support. To my parents, I wish you could have seen my name on a book. I hope that wherever you are, it makes you smile to know that there's an author in the family. Aunt Beverly, thank you for reading my books and sending copies to the grandkids. Michael and Andrew, thanks for your encouragement and lifelong friendship. To my children, you are my heart and my inspiration. And to my husband, Bob, thank you for joining me on this incredible journey called life.

About the Authors

About Felice Gersh, M.D.

Felice Gersh, M.D. is a multi-award winning physician with dual board certifications in OB-GYN and Integrative Medicine. She is the founder and director of the Integrative Medical Group of Irvine, a practice that provides comprehensive health care for women by combining the best evidence-based therapies from conventional, naturopathic, and holistic medicine.

An active part of the PCOS community, Dr. Gersh works with the PCOS Awareness Association and is a member of the PCOS Challenge's Medical/ Scientific Advisory Board. She speaks at the annual conferences of both non-profit organizations. She is a member of the AE-PCOS Society, and has spoken multiple times at their prestigious academic meetings.

She taught obstetrics and gynecology at Keck USC School of Medicine for 12 years as an Assistant Clinical Professor, where she received the highly coveted Outstanding Volunteer Clinical Faculty Award. She now serves as an Affiliate Faculty Member at the Fellowship in Integrative Medicine, through the University of Arizona School of Medicine, where she lectures and regularly grades the case presentations written by the Fellowship students for their final exams.

Additionally, she is a sought after medical forensic expert and has worked on numerous high profile legal cases.

Felice Gersh, M.D. is a prolific writer and lecturer and has been featured in several films and documentary series, including *The Real Skinny on Fat* with Montel Williams, *Fasting*, and *Fork Your Diet*.

Follow her on Instagram at @dr.felicegersh.

About Alexis Perella

Alexis Perella writes about medicine, education, and design. She loves to make complex topics simple. www.alexisperella.com.